IN VIVO AND *EX VIVO* GENE THERAPY FOR INHERITED AND NON-INHERITED DISORDERS

Edited by **Houria Bachtarzi**

***In Vivo* and *Ex Vivo* Gene Therapy for Inherited and Non-Inherited Disorders**
http://dx.doi.org/10.5772/intechopen.72962
Edited by Houria Bachtarzi

Contributors

Chantelle Ahlenstiel, Vera Klemm, Katherine Ognenovska, Scott Ledger, Stuart Turville, Geoff Symonds, Anthony Kelleher, Gustavo Puras, Jose Luis Pedraz, Nusaiba Hasan, Miriam Sainz, Idoia Gallego, Ilia Villate-Beitia, Tania López, Bryan E. Strauss, Otto Cerqueira, Gissele Rolemberg, Igor Vieira, Lana Marlous, Nadine Gimenez, Otavio Rodrigues, Paulo Roberto Del Valle, Samir Andrade Mendonça, Patrick Iversen, Stephen Hollis Bartelmez, Charles Garcia, Stephen Bartelmez, Jan Wijnholds, Henrique Alves, Chandana Herath, Indu Rajapaksha, Peter Angus, Yves Fromes, Caroline Roques-Fromes, Kenya Kamimura, Takeshi Yokoo, Tsutomu Kanefuji, Takeshi Suda, Shuji Terai

First published in London, United Kingdom, 2019 by IntechOpen
IntechOpen is the global imprint of INTECHOPEN LIMITED, registered in England and Wales, registration number: 11086078, The Shard, 25th floor, 32 London Bridge Street
London, SE19SG – United Kingdom
Printed in Croatia

British Library Cataloguing-in-Publication Data
A catalogue record for this book is available from the British Library

Additional hard copies can be obtained from orders@intechopen.com

In Vivo and *Ex Vivo* Gene Therapy for Inherited and Non-Inherited Disorders, Edited by Houria Bachtarzi
p. cm.
Print ISBN 978-1-78985-717-7
Online ISBN 978-1-78985-718-4

For EU product safety concerns:
IN TECH d.o.o., Prolaz Marije Krucifikse Kozulić 3, 51000 Rijeka, Croatia,
info@intechopen.com or visit our website at intechopen.com.

Meet the editor

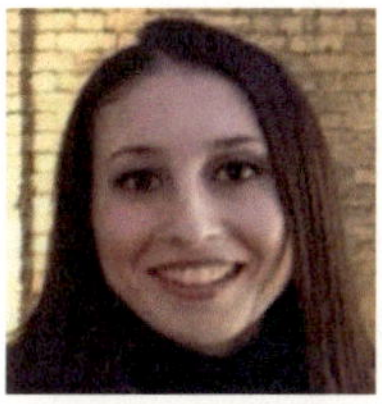

Dr Houria Bachtarzi is a Senior Consultant, Regulatory Affairs - Gene and Cell Therapies, with vast scientific and regulatory experience in the field of advanced biological therapies including virally vectored gene therapy, *in vivo* and *ex vivo* gene editing, cell-based immunotherapy, genetically modified cells for tissue regeneration, genetically engineered immune cells targeting cancer cells, and stem cell-based therapies.
She was previously a Lecturer in Biopharmaceutics and Biotechnology within the Pharmacology and Therapeutics Division at the School of Pharmacy and Biomolecular Sciences, University of Brighton, UK. Houria completed her PhD in cancer gene therapy/viral gene delivery at the University of Oxford, Department of Oncology, followed by Post-Doctoral research work in AAV-based gene therapy and shRNA therapeutics for degenerative neuro-muscular disorders at the Centre for Biomedical Sciences, Royal Holloway-University of London. Houria holds a First Class Master of Pharmacy Degree (with honors) from the University of Bath, UK and is a Registered Pharmacist with the General Pharmaceutical Council in the UK. She is also a Member of the Royal Pharmaceutical Society of Great Britain (RPSGB) and a Member of the British Society for Gene and Cell Therapy (BSGCT). Houria has published a number of peer-reviewed papers in gene therapy and has presented platform presentations at many international and national scientific meetings. In 2014, she received a Rising Star Award from the University of Brighton.

Contents

Preface

Gene therapy constitutes a unique class of advanced biological therapy, which works by transferring genetic materials with the aim of regulating, repairing, replacing, adding, or deleting a genetic sequence of interest. This class encompasses nucleic acids transferred using non-viral systems, recombinant viruses that were modified to express a therapeutic gene of interest, genome editing interventions, and genetically engineered human cells that were modified *ex vivo*.

Over the past decades, gene therapy has seen a massive transformation from a proof-of-concept approach to a clinical reality culminating in the regulatory approval of state-of-the-art products in the European Union and in the United States. These included *in vivo* gene therapy approaches based on recombinant adeno-associated viruses for the treatment of rare inherited genetic disorders such as: lipoprotein lipase deficiency (Glybera®, a replication-deficient adeno-associated virus serotype 1 (AAV1) expressing S447X variant of human lipoprotein lipase (LPL) gene) and retinal dystrophies caused by mutations in the retinal pigment epithelium-specific 65 KDa (RPE65) gene (Luxturna®, a replication-deficient AAV2 expressing human RPE65 gene). Cancer gene therapy has also dominated the scene, with the approval of cutting-edge gene therapy products. These include the first oncolytic virotherapy for melanoma based on attenuated non-integrating Herpes Simplex Virus-1 (HSV-1) modified not only to efficiently replicate within tumors, but also to express the immune stimulatory protein granulocyte macrophage colony-stimulating factor (GM-CSF). Non-solid tumors, notably B-cell acute lymphoblastic leukaemia (ALL), diffuse large B-cell lymphoma (DLBCL), and primary mediastinal large B-cell lymphoma (PMBCL) have also seen progress in their therapeutic management with the approval of a new generation of *ex vivo* autologous genetically modified T-cell based cancer immunotherapies (Kymriah® and Yescarta®, autologous T-cells genetically engineered with a lentiviral vector (used during Kymriah® manufacturing)/retroviral vector (used during Yescarta® manufacturing) to express anti-CD19 chimeric antigen receptor (CAR)). The clinical and marketing authorization successes of these gene/genetically modified cell-based technologies in cancer and rare genetic diseases have now opened up the pathway for gene therapy application in other new target indications including infections and diabetes.

Gene therapy is continuously shaping and revolutionizing the field of medicine, with more cutting-edge therapies including genome editing-based medicines entering the clinic and becoming a treatment modality in the next 5-10 years.

This book captures some of the scientific progresses notably in gene transfer technologies as well the preclinical and clinical developments of gene therapy interventions (both *ex vivo* and *in vivo*) in the treatment of a broad range of debilitating inherited and non-inherited genetic disorders.

Houria Bachtarzi, DPhil (Oxon), MPharm (Hons), MRPharmS
ERA Consulting (UK) Ltd
A member of the ERA Consulting Group of Companies
London Gas Museum, Twelvetrees Crescent
London, United Kingdom

Section 1

Gene Transfer Technologies for *In Vivo* and *Ex Vivo* Applications

Chapter 1

Nucleic Acid-Based Therapy: Development of a Nonviral-Based Delivery Approach

Takeshi Yokoo, Kenya Kamimura, Tsutomu Kanefuji,
Takeshi Suda and Shuji Terai

Additional information is available at the end of the chapter

http://dx.doi.org/10.5772/intechopen.80741

Abstract

Gene therapy returns to the center stage of medicine to treat patients with diseases that are unable to be cured with the conventional therapeutic strategies. This development is due to various reasons, including vector development and significant achievement in next-generation sequencing. Among the various methodologies of gene therapy, nucleic acid-based therapy has been considered to be promising in various diseases. The development of delivery methods to target cells *in vivo*, however, remains critical. These include viral vector-based and nonviral vector-based gene delivery methods as well as physical approaches such as hydrodynamic gene delivery (HGD). HGD is a simple and effective *in vivo* gene transfer method for the functional analysis of therapeutic genes and regulatory elements in small animals. Moreover, this chapter outlines the principle of HGD, gene expression studies in rodents, and recent advances in clinical application of HGD and provides future perspectives in developing a safe and efficient method for nucleic acid-based therapy.

Keywords: nucleic acid-based therapy, nonviral delivery, hydrodynamic gene delivery, site-specificity, computer-controlled injection, human gene therapy

1. Introduction

In 1990, first human gene therapy was conducted, targeting adenosine deaminase deficiency *via* retrovirus-mediated delivery system [1]. Since then, the number of clinical trials has gradually increased, and approximately 2600 trials have been globally undertaken or approved until November 2017 [2]. Most trials (75%) utilized a viral vector as a delivery tool of gene. Viral vector-based delivery resulted in a high level of gene expression for a long period;

however, carcinogenesis and lethal immune reaction were reported [3–5]. Numerous researchers have been attempting to overcome these serious obstacles to enable safe and efficient therapy. For this purpose, the improvement of viral vector has been extensively studied in the last decade, and in addition, nonviral vector-based gene delivery method has developed with great promise. As expected, it resulted in less antigenicity and less chance of integration into the human genome than viral vector; therefore, it can be regarded as a biologically safer method than viral vector-based gene delivery method. However, the period of transgene expression tends to be limited.

This chapter focuses on nonviral vector-based delivery method, which could be used for the nucleic acid-based therapy. In these methods, a transgene is not integrated into the host genome; hence, gene expression is transient. Because temporal transgene expression is applied to promising technologies, such as generation of iPS cells and gene editing by CRISPR/Cas9, nonviral vector-based gene delivery may play a big role in future medicine.

The last section of this chapter outlines the recent progress in the HGD, which enables the highest level of delivery efficiency among nonviral vector-based approaches and the clinical application utilizing the well-established method of catheter insertion into the vessels in the multiple organs.

2. Nonviral approaches for nucleic acid transfer

This section focuses on gene delivery methods using nonviral vector-based approach. Nucleic acids loaded in artificial or natural cargos or in naked condition are transferred to target cells. The characteristics of various gene deliveries are briefly described in **Table 1**.

2.1. Liposome-based approach

Lipofection, a cationic lipid-mediated approach, is widely used in numerous *in vitro* and *in vivo* studies. The first study reporting lipofection was published in 1987 [6]. Molecules comprising hydrophilic head, linker, and hydrophobic anchor form a spherical structure. The positively charged hydrophilic head plays a role in condensing the negatively charged DNAs. It also helps in establishing an electrostatic interaction with the negatively charged cell membrane. As a result, it promotes the cellular uptake of DNA-loaded liposome (lipoplex), endosomal escape, and subsequent release of the condensed DNAs into the cytoplasm. On the contrary, the hydrophobic anchor protects DNAs from degradation by nucleases. Liposome is a popular carrier to deliver even large-sized transgene; it is easy to prepare and modify and is utilized in numerous laboratories worldwide. Nevertheless, there are several drawbacks for its use in gene therapy. It has difficulty in achieving therapeutic level of transgene expression, shows no tropism to desired cells, and exhibits a short life span. Furthermore, the positively charged head has cell toxicity. An inflammatory response occurs when unmethylated CpG DNA is transported, which is one of the obstacles that need to be addressed. Various strategies to achieve high level of safety and efficiency, such as introduction and improvement of polyethylene

Method	Functional component	Advantages	Disadvantages
Lipids	Cationic lipids	High efficiency *in vitro* Ease to prepare	Low efficiency *in vivo* Acute immune response
Polymers	Cationic polymers	Highly effective *in vitro* Ease to prepare	Toxic to cells Acute immune response
Exosomes	Natural or modified exosomes	Less toxic (Insufficient data)	Low efficiency? (Insufficient data)
Needle injection	Mechanic force	Simple	Low efficiency Expression limited to needle track
Gene gun	Pressure	Good efficiency	Limited to target area Need surgical procedure for internal organ
Electroporation	Electric pulse	High efficiency	Tissue damage Limited target area Need surgical procedure for internal organ
Sonoporation	Ultrasound	Site specific	Low efficiency Tissue damage
Magnetofection	Magnetic field	Site specific	Low efficiency Limited target area Need surgical procedure for internal organ
Hydrodynamic delivery	Hydrodynamic pressure	Simple High efficiency Site specific	Need catheter insertion technique in large animals

Table 1. Characteristics of nonviral gene delivery method.

glycol [7] and cell-specific targeting ligand on the surface of the liposome, have been extensively studied. Development of a promising linker also improves stability, biodegradability, and transfection efficiency and reduces cytotoxicity [8]. Lipofection has been utilized in 4.4% of clinical trials worldwide [2]. The results of human gene therapy for cystic fibrosis in clinical trials of phase I/IIa and IIb have been reported in the UK [9, 10]. Patients had cystic fibrosis transmembrane conductance regulator (CFTR) gene mutations and suffered from hypofunction of CFTR in multiple organs. Because secretory fluid becomes viscous, the patient may experience repeated respiratory infection and, finally, respiratory failure. CFTR gene was nebulized as lipoplex every 28 days for 1 year for significant stabilization of lung function [9, 10]. In 2016, other clinical trials for genitourinary cancers and solid tumors reportedly used the truncated forms of the RB gene and p53 gene with docetaxel, respectively [11, 12].

2.2. Polymer-based approach

Cationic polymer is an artificially synthesized vehicle, and various types of polymer have been studied. DNA condensed in cationic polymer (polyplex) acquires tolerance to enzymatic degradation, which results in stability in the blood. Cellular uptake is via receptor-mediated endocytosis, which leads to a high level of transfection activity. Clinical trials using this approach for cystic fibrosis and ocular degenerative disease have been reported [13, 14]. Nevertheless, the stability of polyplex and persistent positive charge leads to high cytotoxicity.

Because cationic polymer is easy to prepare and improve, various constructs, such as polyethylenimine, polyamidoamine, polyallylamine, chitosan, dendrimers, cationic proteins, and peptides, have been studied to overcome the obstacles.

2.3. Lipopolyplex-based approach

Lipopolyplex comprises polycation (cationic polymer or peptide) and condensed DNA with lipid shell and is divided into diverse categories according to the combination and ternary structure. Its advantages are of both lipoplex and polyplex, that is, more efficient transfection and less cytotoxicity. Previous study [15] and reviews [16, 17] have described the strategy, variety, and preparation of lipopolyplex.

2.4. Exosome-based approach

Exosome is a kind of extracellular vesicle secreted by various cells. It comprises a lipid bilayer with several surface antigens derived from the parent cell. DNA, mRNA, miRNA, and protein can be included in the lipid bilayer. Moreover, exosome is known to have organ and cell tropism; however, the mechanism is not completely clarified. This indicates that exosome plays a role in intercellular communication. Cancer cells as well as healthy cells secrete exosome. Integrin included in exosome reportedly determines organ tropism for metastasis. Exosome from metastatic lung tumor of breast cancer induced lung metastasis of breast cancer, which originally had metastatic ability only to the bone [18]. An attempt to utilize cancer-derived exosome for cancer therapy was also reported, wherein the cancer-derived exosome was used as a natural carrier of CRISPR/Cas9 plasmids. Compared to epithelial cell-derived exosome, cancer-derived exosome with CRISPR/Cas9 plasmids selectively accumulated in cancer cells, suppressed PARP-1 gene expression, and achieved induction of apoptosis [19]. Recently, many researchers have been studying exosome as delivery system for cancer therapy. Surface antigens of exosomes are known to be modified directly and genetically. The exosomes from leukemia cells, marrow stromal cells, adipose-derived mesenchymal stem cells, breast cancer cells, and kidney cells including siRNA and miRNA were reported to be used for colorectal tumor, glioma, hepatocellular carcinoma, breast cancer, and chronic myelogenous leukemia [20–24]. Although the exosome-based approach has been seen as a new and promising method of gene delivery, it is rather obvious that further understandings of the mechanisms and structures as well as improvement in exosomes' preparation are necessary to achieve the high level of efficiency and safety needed for clinical application.

2.5. Needle injection

Direct injection to the tissue is the simplest approach for the physical delivery of nucleic acid. The first report for delivery to muscle was published in 1990 [25]. Needle injection was expanded to the skin [26], heart muscle [27], liver [28], and tumor [29]. Currently, microneedle is studied as a minimally invasive delivery for skin disease and vaccination [30, 31]. Microneedles are arrays of 25–2000-μm long needles [32]; on the basis of the delivery mechanism, they are divided into solid, coated, and dissolving types [31]. In a mouse study, siRNA delivery is reported to be effective for skin conditions with aberrant gene expression, such as alopecia, allergic skin diseases, hyperpigmentation, psoriasis, skin cancer, and congenital pachyonychia [33].

2.6. Gene gun

Gene gun is known as microprojectile bombardment, and the first study reporting its use was published in 1987 [34]. At first, this method was developed for gene delivery into plant cells. A bullet with the microparticles containing DNA is shot to a target cell, and gene delivery is achieved. On the basis of the principle of obtaining a driving force, a gene gun is divided into three major groups: powder gene gun [34], high-voltage electric gene gun [35], and gas gene gun [36]. The driving force moves the microparticles containing DNA toward a target tissue and penetrates the cell membrane. Because delivery efficiency and cell damage are two sides of the same coin, appropriate operating pressure is required. A phase I clinical study was performed to treat melanoma using *IL-12* gene [37]. Although an attempt of combining delivery with microneedles reportedly enhanced the penetration depths of microparticles [38], gene gun may be more appropriate for delivery to the skin, such as for vaccination.

2.7. Sonoporation, electroporation, and magnetofection

Sonoporation, using ultrasound [39, 40], and electroporation, using electric pulse [41], increase the permeability of cell membrane for cellular uptake of nucleic acid. Magnetofection utilizes magnetic field to enable microparticles with nucleic acid to pass through the cell membrane [42]. These methods are used in combination with other methods, such as lipofection, to protect nucleic acid against degradation by nucleases. To increase gene delivery efficiency of sonoporation, microbubbles were shown to be effective [43] and applied for delivery to cancer cells [44, 45] and the central nervous system [46, 47]. Clinical trials in phases I and II have been reported for the treatment of melanoma [48–50] and solid tumors [51].

2.8. Hydrodynamic gene delivery (HGD)

HGD is one of the simplest methods for gene transfer. The efficiency of HGD is the highest among nonviral vector-based delivery methods, and its physical force to deliver the gene into the cells relies on a high level of flow rate and volume of the injected solution. Since the first published reports in 1999 [52, 53], many researchers have utilized this methodology for gene transfer in animal experiments, particularly in rodent studies. For its application in human, safety and efficacy of this approach have been extensively studied and improved. To date, various types of nucleic acid have been delivered by this approach in rodents as well as pigs [54–57], dogs [58, 59], and rhesus monkeys [60, 61]. Functional analyses of therapeutic gene were reported in nonalcoholic steatohepatitis [62], hepatitis B and C [63], fulminant hepatitis [64, 65], liver fibrosis [66, 67], liver regeneration [68], Fabry's disease [64], and colon cancer [69]. The next section describes its principle and progress in human gene therapy.

3. Principle and progress of hydrodynamic gene delivery toward human gene therapy

3.1. Principle, efficiency, and safety of hydrodynamic gene delivery

HGD is achieved by the quick injection of a large amount of naked nucleic acid solution into the vein. In case of a rodent, the solution is injected from the tail vein. The most important step of successful gene delivery is a precise insertion of an injection needle into the tail vein. The details of technical tips are described in **Figure 1**. The quick injection can transiently increase an intravenous pressure. Mechanical force by rapid increase in venous pressure allows nucleic acid to pass through the cell membrane into the cytoplasm and nucleus.

Among various organs, the liver can achieve the highest level of gene expression because of the presence of the specific structure fenestra. Fenestra is a small window in the sinusoidal vessel, and hepatocytes are partly exposed to the blood stream. In other words, hepatocytes can be directly affected by intravascular pressure. A rapid stream of hydrodynamic injection can wash out the blood in the sinusoid vessel transiently and thoroughly, and nucleic acid can reach the hepatocytes without degeneration by nucleases. A high intravascular pressure

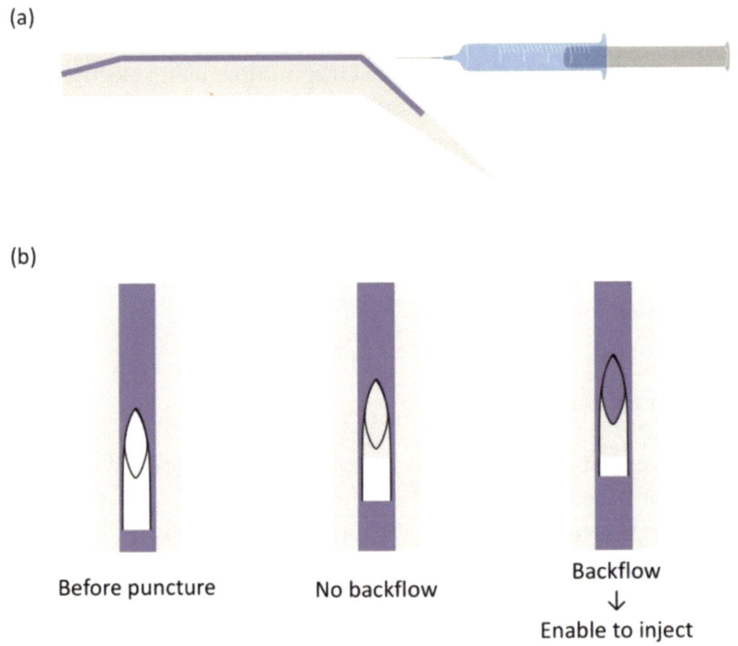

Figure 1. Technical details of the tail vein injection in a mouse. (a) When inserting a needle tip, the tail vein and needle shaft should be at the same angle. The puncture can be performed from the top of the tail curve. (b) If a needle tip successfully enters the tail vein, backflow of the blood is visible on the needle tip. Once the backflow is confirmed, a needle tip can be further inserted to the proximal side of the tail vein.

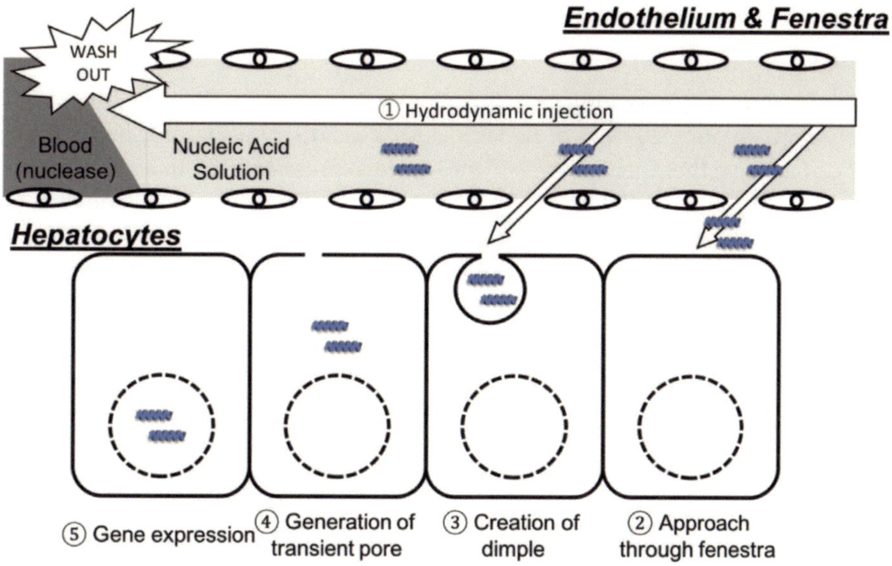

Figure 2. Scheme of hydrodynamic gene delivery. The hepatocyte partly faces to the blood stream via the fenestra in the sinusoidal structure. A rapid stream of hydrodynamic injection has the blood in the sinusoid washed out transiently, and the nucleic acid can be delivered into hepatocytes without being degraded by nucleases. A high intravascular pressure makes dimples on the surface of hepatocyte, and finally generates transient pores. Nucleic acid is pushed into the hepatocyte through the transient pores.

creates dimples on the surface of the hepatocyte and finally generates transient small pores. The nucleic acid is pushed into the hepatocyte through the transient pores **(Figure 2)**. Moreover, it was clarified that the pores naturally reduce and disappear in 24–48 h [70]. Although serum transaminase shows transient increase after a hydrodynamic injection, these values return to the background level within a short period. Considering the short life time of transaminase, an increase in serum transaminase is speculated to be caused by leakage from the transient pores. If the intravascular pressure is kept within an adequate range, this change in hepatocyte is reversible and does not result in apoptosis and necrosis; therefore, acute liver failure is not a concern.

To apply this method into the clinic, the modification of the original procedure is essential as in mouse studies, hydrodynamic injection is performed via the tail vein. Looking back to the original method, in detail, naked DNA solution equivalent to 10% of the body weight (BW) is injected for 5–7 s via the tail vein. The details of hydrodynamics during the injection have been reported using contrast medium under fluoroscopic imaging and cone-beam computed tomography (CT) [71]. Briefly, the injected solution is led to the inferior vena cava (IVC) and then flowed back to the hepatic veins. The retrograde flow passes through the sinusoid vessel into the portal vein. Given that contrast medium transiently stayed in the liver after the injection, the flow generated transient pores on the surface of the hepatocyte while passing through the sinusoid vessel. Because of the filling of sinusoidal and interstitial space by the solution and transfer of nucleic acid into the hepatocyte, the volume of the liver reportedly increased by 165% compared to the preinjected condition.

The efficiency of transfer was indicated by microscopic images. Transgene expression was observed in approximately 20–40% of hepatocytes. Wide distribution of transgene expression in the liver can achieve therapeutic level of transgene expression [72]. In a rat model with bile duct ligation, hydrodynamic delivery of MMP13 gene indicated prophylactic effect on liver fibrosis [67]. Given its simplicity, safety, and efficiency, HGD has been utilized in numerous rodent studies [63, 65, 66, 73, 74]. HGD can be also applied to various organs other than the liver, such as the kidneys [75], muscle [61], and pancreas [76].

3.2. Improvement of a hydrodynamic injection for larger animals

Based on efficiency and safety in rodents, HGD has been improved extensively and can be potentially applied in humans **(Figure 3)**. Two major obstacles that should be overcome are poor site specificity and very large injection volume. HGD with adequate range of intravascular pressure, a key factor for efficient and safe delivery, is facile to achieve by a manual injection in mice. On the contrary, in larger animals, such as rabbits, pigs, dogs, and nonhuman primates, controlling intravascular pressure is difficult because of a large amount of injection

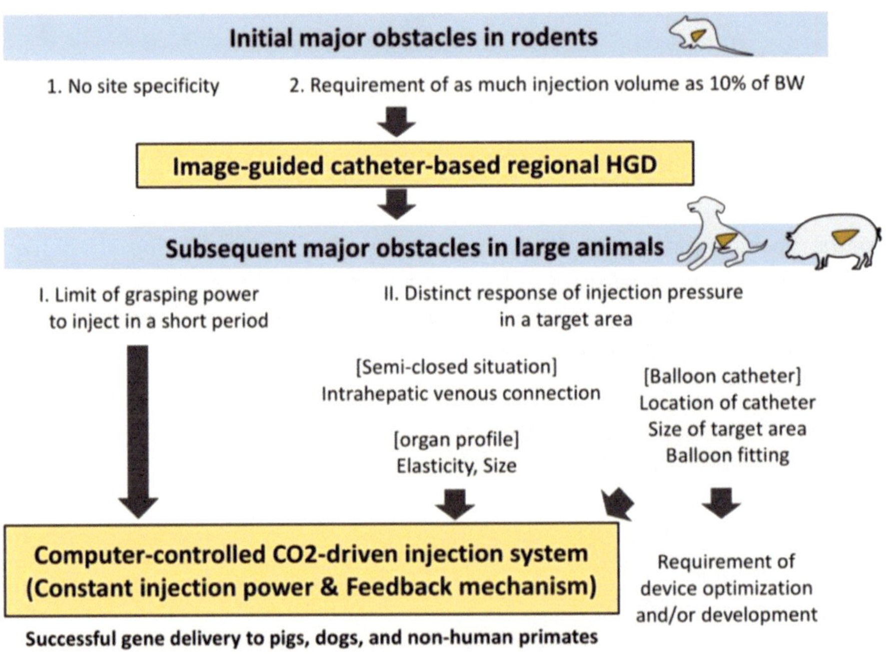

Figure 3. Improvements of hydrodynamic gene delivery toward human gene therapy.

volume per second. Several studies have tried to resolve these problems using catheter technique. A balloon catheter is inserted from the jugular vein into the hepatic vein under X-ray guidance, which is often performed in clinic [56]. When the catheter is placed in the hepatic vein, the balloon on its tip is inflated, which causes venous occlusion to prevent leakage of DNA solution from the hepatic vein to the IVC. This technique targeting each lobe of the liver can reduce injection volume per one procedure to <1% BW, maintaining efficiency of gene delivery.

During the establishment of catheter technique, another important problem arises, that is, distinct response of injection pressure in a targeted area. Precise control of intravascular pressure is essential to achieve efficient and safe gene delivery (**Figure 4**). Inconsistent intravascular pressure caused by leakage of DNA solution to the adjacent area, which results from physiological connections of intrahepatic vessels and tissue elasticity, is highly possible, and the leakage volume can be also associated with intravascular pressure during injection. To achieve precise control of intravascular pressure, a computer-controlled injector with feedback mechanism has been developed [54]. Although the initial version of the injector utilized CO_2 as its driving force, the current version adopts electric motor for pursuit of more accurate control [58, 77] (**Figure 5**). This injection system leads to reproducible results of efficiency. Not only efficiency but also safety is confirmed in various aspects, such as blood test, electrocardiogram, hemodynamic CT study, laparoscopic observation, and histologic assessment [56, 78, 79] (**Figure 6**).

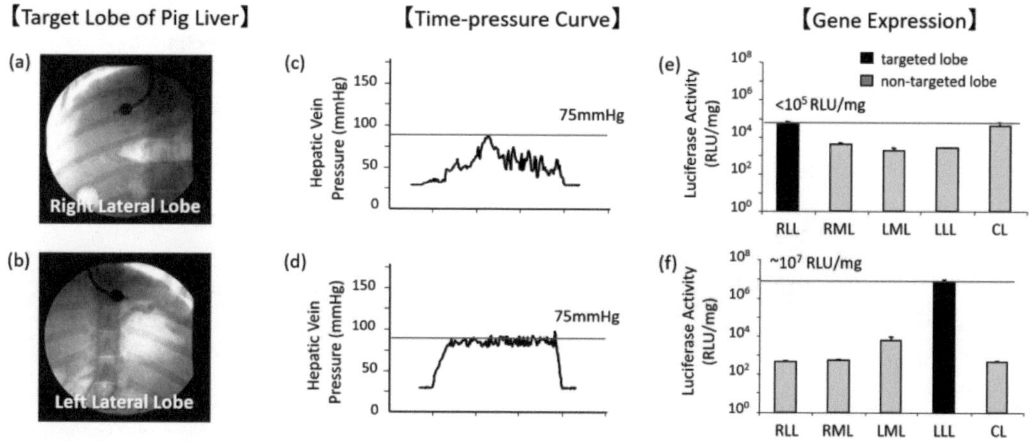

Figure 4. Relationship between time-pressure curve and transgene expression on site-specific delivery to a large animal. (a and b) HGD was performed to right and left lateral lobes of the pig liver. (c and d) Both injections achieved 75 mmHg of a peak intravascular pressure. (e and f) Gene expressions after the injections of (c) and (d) are shown in (e) and (f), respectively. This figure is partly reused and modified with updated information from Figures 3, 5, and 6 in [56] with their permission. RLL, right lateral lobe; RML, right medial lobe; LML, left medial lobe; LLL, left lateral lobe; CL, caudate lobe.

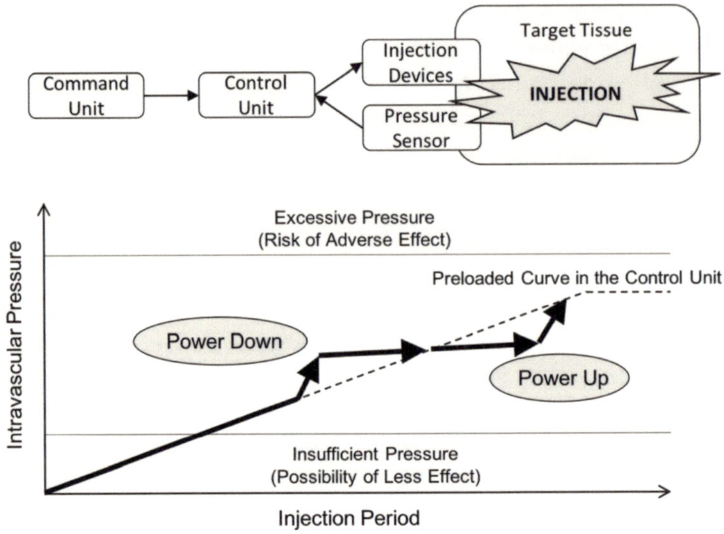

Figure 5. Scheme of the computer-controlled hydrodynamic injection system. Prior to an injection, a user selects appropriate time-pressure pattern for delivery and preload the data to the command unit. The command unit transmits the data to the control unit, which modulates electric power based on the feedback information of an intravascular pressure during the injection from the pressure sensor placed at the peripheral vein of a target area.

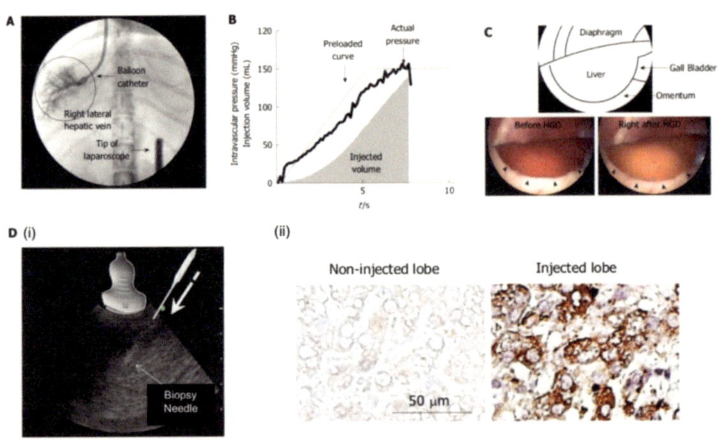

Figure 6. Image-guided, computer-controlled HGD to the dog liver. The balloon catheter was placed at the appropriate position in the hepatic veins of right lateral lobe and the occlusion of the blood flow by the balloon was confirmed by injecting a small amount of contrast medium into the hepatic vein. Then the hydrodynamic injection of naked DNA solution was performed under the real time monitoring of liver structure by the laparoscope using the computer-controlled injection system (A). (B) Time-pressure curve and the volume of injected solution recorded in the injection system. Solid and dotted lines represent actual and preloaded time-pressure curves. The gray area shows cumulative volume of injected saline (ml). (C) Laparoscopic findings of the hydrodynamically injected right lateral lobe of the dog. The injected lobe was swollen, and the injected DNA solution transiently made the liver pale. Neither destruction nor bleeding was seen on the surface of the liver (arrowheads). (D) The effect of lobe-specific hydrodynamic gene delivery of luciferase expressing plasmid. (i) Liver samples were collected by needle biopsy under the ultrasound sonography 4 days after the injection. (ii) The immunohistochemical analyses showed positively stained cells in the injected right lateral lobe. No stained cells were found in noninjected left lateral lobe. This figure is partly reused and modified with updated information from Figure 1 in [58] with their permission.

4. Conclusion

Currently, various approaches including both viral and nonviral vector-based delivery methods are studied for safe and efficient human gene therapy. They have their own properties, such as duration of gene expression, size of transgene to load, possible organs and their expected volumes in single procedure, and repeatability. Conditions to treat are also diverse. Congenital disease such as hemophilia possibly requires long-term transgene expression for decades. For *in vivo* gene editing based on CRISPR/Cas9, short-term transgene expression may be preferred, to prevent off-target effect. Therefore, the transient gene expression mediated by the nonviral vector-based delivery may have great advantages when it comes to gene editing. Among the methods, as described above, HGD may be a promising delivery approach as it is simpler and more efficient. Currently, we are modifying the original HGD method used in small animals in order to apply it into large animals to test its efficacy and safety. Metabolic and genetic diseases, which show lower level of normal functional protein, are so far good candidates for this type of procedure. Although there is evidence showing transgene expression and that the procedure was safely performed in pigs [54–57], dogs [58, 59], and baboons [60, 61], further preclinical studies are necessary prior to human therapy application.

Acknowledgements

This work was supported in part by grant-in-aid for scientific research from the Japanese Society for the Promotion of Sciences, 16K19333 to Yokoo T, 17K09408 to Kamimura.

This work has finished due to Dexi Liu, and all members at Division of Gastroenterology and Hepatology, Graduate School of Medical and Dental Sciences, Niigata University. The authors would like to appreciate all members at the Niigata city industrial promotion center and for their excellent assistance in producing the system, Yoshihiko Ohba for the supporting of fine-tuning of the system.

Conflict of interest

The authors declare no conflict of interest.

Author details

Takeshi Yokoo[1,2], Kenya Kamimura[2*], Tsutomu Kanefuji[3], Takeshi Suda[3] and Shuji Terai[2]

*Address all correspondence to: kenya-k@med.niigata-u.ac.jp

1 Department of Preemptive Medicine for Digestive Diseases and Healthy Active Life, Niigata University School of Medicine, Chuo-ku, Niigata, Japan

2 Division of Gastroenterology and Hepatology, Graduate School of Medical and Dental Sciences, Niigata University, Chuo-ku, Niigata, Japan

3 Department of Gastroenterology and Hepatology, Institute of Community Medicine, Niigata University Medical and Dental Hospital, Minamiuonuma, Niigata, Japan

References

[1] Blaese RM, Culver KW, Miller AD, et al. T lymphocyte-directed gene therapy for ADA- SCID: Initial trial results after 4 years. Science. 1995;**270**:475-480. DOI: 10.1126/science.270.5235.475

[2] Ginn SL, Amaya AK, Alexander IE, et al. Gene therapy clinical trials worldwide to 2017: An update. The Journal of Gene Medicine. 2018;**20**:e3015. DOI: 10.1002/jgm.3015

[3] Hacein-Bey-Abina S, Von Kalle C, Schmidt M, et al. LMO2-associated clonal T cell proliferation in two patients after gene therapy for SCID-X1. Science. 2003;**302**:415-419. DOI: 10.1126/science.1088547

[4] Manno CS, Pierce GF, Arruda VR, et al. Successful transduction of liver in hemophilia by AAV-Factor IX and limitations imposed by the host immune response. Nature Medicine. 2006;**12**:342-347. DOI: 10.1038/nm1358

[5] Howe SJ, Mansour MR, Schwarzwaelder K, et al. Insertional mutagenesis in combination with acquired somatic mutations leads to leukemogenesis following gene therapy of SCID-X1. The Journal of Clinical Investigation. 2008;**44**:1-22. DOI: 10.1172/JCI35798DS1

[6] Felgner PL, Gadek TR, Holm M, et al. Lipofection: A highly efficient, lipid-mediated DNA-transfection procedure. Proceedings of the National Academy of Sciences of the United States of America. 1987;**84**:7413-7417

[7] Dong H, Tang M, Li Y, et al. Disulfide-bridged cleavable PEGylation in polymeric nanomedicine for controlled therapeutic delivery. Nanomedicine (London, England). 2015;**10**:1941-1958. DOI: 10.2217/nnm.15.38

[8] Zhi D, Bai Y, Yang J, et al. A review on cationic lipids with different linkers for gene delivery. Advances in Colloid and Interface Science. 2018;**253**:117-140. DOI: 10.1016/j.cis.2017.12.006

[9] Alton EWFW, Boyd AC, Porteous DJ, et al. A phase I/IIa safety and efficacy study of nebulized liposome-mediated gene therapy for cystic fibrosis supports a multidose trial. American Journal of Respiratory and Critical Care Medicine. 2015;**192**:1389-1392. DOI: 10.1164/rccm.201506-1193LE

[10] Alton EWFW, Armstrong DK, Ashby D, et al. Repeated nebulisation of non-viral CFTR gene therapy in patients with cystic fibrosis: A randomised, double-blind, placebo-controlled, phase 2b trial. The Lancet Respiratory Medicine. 2015;**3**:684-691. DOI: 10.1016/S2213-2600(15)00245-3

[11] Siefker-Radtke A, Zhang X, Guo CC, et al. A phase 1 study of a tumor-targeted systemic nanodelivery system, SGT-94, in genitourinary cancers. Molecular Therapy. 2016;**24**:1484-1491. DOI: 10.1038/mt.2016.118

[12] Pirollo KF, Nemunaitis J, Leung PK, et al. Safety and efficacy in advanced solid tumors of a targeted nanocomplex carrying the p53 gene used in combination with docetaxel: A phase 1b study. Molecular Therapy. 2016;**24**:1697-1706. DOI: 10.1038/mt.2016.135

[13] Konstan MW, Davis PB, Wagener JS, et al. Compacted DNA nanoparticles administered to the nasal mucosa of cystic fibrosis subjects are safe and demonstrate partial to complete cystic fibrosis transmembrane regulator reconstitution. Human Gene Therapy. 2004;**15**: 1255-1269. DOI: 10.1089/hum.2004.15.1255

[14] Sweeney P, Karashima T, Ishikura H, et al. Efficient therapeutic gene delivery after systemic administration of a novel polyethylenimine/DNA vector in an orthotopic bladder cancer model. Cancer Research. 2003;**63**:4017-4020

[15] Chen W, Li H, Liu Z, et al. Lipopolyplex for therapeutic gene delivery and its application for the treatment of Parkinson's disease. Frontiers in Aging Neuroscience. 2016;**8**:68. DOI: 10.3389/fnagi.2016.00068

[16] Hadinoto K, Sundaresan A, Cheow WS. Lipid–polymer hybrid nanoparticles as a new generation therapeutic delivery platform: A review. European Journal of Pharmaceutics and Biopharmaceutics. 2013;**85**:427-443. DOI: 10.1016/j.ejpb.2013.07.002

[17] Rezaee M, Oskuee RK, Nassirli H, et al. Progress in the development of lipopolyplexes as efficient non-viral gene delivery systems. Journal of Controlled Release. 2016;**236**:1-14. DOI: 10.1016/j.jconrel.2016.06.023

[18] Hoshino A, Costa-Silva B, Shen T-L, et al. Tumour exosome integrins determine organotropic metastasis. Nature. 2015;**527**:329-335. DOI: 10.1038/nature15756

[19] Kim SM, Yang Y, Oh SJ, et al. Cancer-derived exosomes as a delivery platform of CRISPR/Cas9 confer cancer cell tropism-dependent targeting. Journal of Controlled Release. 2017; **266**:8-16. DOI: 10.1016/j.jconrel.2017.09.013

[20] Akao Y, Nakagawa Y, Hirata I, et al. Role of anti-oncomirs miR-143 and -145 in human colorectal tumors. Cancer Gene Therapy. 2010;**17**:398-408. DOI: 10.1038/cgt.2009.88

[21] Katakowski M, Buller B, Zheng X, et al. Exosomes from marrow stromal cells expressing miR-146b inhibit glioma growth. Cancer Letters. 2013;**335**:201-204. DOI: 10.1016/j.canlet.2013.02.019

[22] Lou G, Song X, Yang F, et al. Exosomes derived from miR-122-modified adipose tissue-derived MSCs increase chemosensitivity of hepatocellular carcinoma. Journal of Hematology & Oncology. 2015;**8**:122. DOI: 10.1186/s13045-015-0220-7

[23] O'Brien K, Lowry MC, Corcoran C, et al. miR-134 in extracellular vesicles reduces triple-negative breast cancer aggression and increases drug sensitivity. Oncotarget. 2015;**6**: 32774-32789. DOI: 10.18632/oncotarget.5192

[24] Bellavia D, Raimondo S, Calabrese G, et al. Interleukin 3- receptor targeted exosomes inhibit *in vitro* and *in vivo* Chronic Myelogenous Leukemia cell growth. Theranostics. 2017;**7**:1333-1345. DOI: 10.7150/thno.17092

[25] Wolff JA, Malone RW, Williams P, et al. Direct gene transfer into mouse muscle in vivo. Science. 1990;**247**:1465-1468

[26] Choate KA, Khavari PA. Direct cutaneous gene delivery in a human genetic skin disease. Human Gene Therapy. 1997;**8**:1659-1665. DOI: 10.1089/hum.1997.8.14-1659

[27] Park SW, Gwon HC, Jeong JO, et al. Intracardiac echocardiographic guidance and monitoring during percutaneous endomyocardial gene injection in porcine heart. Human Gene Therapy. 2001;**12**:893-903. DOI: 10.1089/104303401750195863

[28] Hickman MA, Malone RW, Lehmann-Bruinsma K, et al. Gene expression following direct injection of DNA into liver. Human Gene Therapy. 1994;**5**:1477-1483. DOI: 10.1089/hum.1994.5.12-1477

[29] Habib NA, Ding SF, el-Masry R, et al. Preliminary report: The short-term effects of direct p53 DNA injection in primary hepatocellular carcinomas. Cancer Detection and Prevention. 1996;**20**:103-107

[30] McLean WHI, Moore CBT. Keratin disorders: From gene to therapy. Human Molecular Genetics. 2011;**20**:R189-R197. DOI: 10.1093/hmg/ddr379

[31] Chen W, Li H, Shi D, et al. Microneedles as a delivery system for gene therapy. Frontiers in Pharmacology. 2016;**7**:137. DOI: 10.3389/fphar.2016.00137

[32] Donnelly RF, Singh TRR, Woolfson AD. Microneedle-based drug delivery systems: Microfabrication, drug delivery, and safety. Drug Delivery. 2010;**17**:187-207. DOI: 10.3109/10717541003667798

[33] Deng Y, Chen J, Zhao Y, et al. Transdermal delivery of siRNA through microneedle array. Scientific Reports. 2016;**6**:21422. DOI: 10.1038/srep21422

[34] Klein TM, Wolf ED, Wu R, et al. High-velocity microprojectiles for delivering nucleic acids into living cells. Nature. 1987;**327**:70-73. DOI: 10.1038/327070a0

[35] Christou P, McCabe DE, Martinell BJ, et al. Soybean genetic engineering—Commercial production of transgenic plants. Trends in Biotechnology. 1990;**8**:145-151. DOI: 10.1016/0167-7799(90)90160-Y

[36] Soliman SM, Abdallah S, Gutmark E, et al. Numerical simulation of microparticles penetration and gas dynamics in an axi-symmetric supersonic nozzle for genetic vaccination. Powder Technology. 2011;**208**:676-683. DOI: 10.1016/J.POWTEC.2011.01.008

[37] Sun Y, Jurgovsky K, Möller P, et al. Vaccination with IL-12 gene-modified autologous melanoma cells: Preclinical results and a first clinical phase I study. Gene Therapy. 1998;**5**:481-490. DOI: 10.1038/sj.gt.3300619

[38] Zhang D, Das DB, Rielly CD. An experimental study of microneedle-assisted microparticle delivery. Journal of Pharmaceutical Sciences. 2013;**102**:3632-3644. DOI: 10.1002/jps.23665

[39] Kim HJ, Greenleaf JF, Kinnick RR, et al. Ultrasound-mediated transfection of mammalian cells. Human Gene Therapy. 1996;**7**:1339-1346. DOI: 10.1089/hum.1996.7.11-1339

[40] Miao CH, Brayman AA, Loeb KR, et al. Ultrasound enhances gene delivery of human factor IX plasmid. Human Gene Therapy. 2005;**16**:893-905. DOI: 10.1089/hum.2005.16.893

[41] Neumann E, Schaefer-Ridder M, Wang Y, et al. Gene transfer into mouse lyoma cells by electroporation in high electric fields. The EMBO Journal. 1982;**1**:841-845

[42] Plank C, Anton M, Rudolph C, et al. Enhancing and targeting nucleic acid delivery by magnetic force. Expert Opinion on Biological Therapy. 2003;**3**:745-758. DOI: 10.1517/14712598.3.5.745

[43] Lawrie A, Brisken A, Francis S, et al. Microbubble-enhanced ultrasound for vascular gene delivery. Gene Therapy. 2000;**7**:2023-2027. DOI: 10.1038/sj.gt.3301339

[44] Chang S, Guo J, Sun J, et al. Targeted microbubbles for ultrasound mediated gene transfection and apoptosis induction in ovarian cancer cells. Ultrasonics Sonochemistry. 2013;**20**:171-179. DOI: 10.1016/j.ultsonch.2012.06.015

[45] Ji Y, Han Z, Shao L, et al. Evaluation of in vivo antitumor effects of low-frequency ultrasound-mediated miRNA-133a microbubble delivery in breast cancer. Cancer Medicine. 2016;**5**:2534-2543. DOI: 10.1002/cam4.840

[46] Tan J-KY, Pham B, Zong Y, et al. Microbubbles and ultrasound increase intraventricular polyplex gene transfer to the brain. Journal of Controlled Release. 2016;**231**:86-93. DOI: 10.1016/j.jconrel.2016.02.003

[47] Song Z, Wang Z, Shen J, et al. Nerve growth factor delivery by ultrasound-mediated nanobubble destruction as a treatment for acute spinal cord injury in rats. International Journal of Nanomedicine. 2017;**12**:1717-1729. DOI: 10.2147/IJN.S128848

[48] Wilgenhof S, Corthals J, Heirman C, et al. Phase II study of autologous monocyte-derived mRNA electroporated dendritic cells (TriMixDC-MEL) plus ipilimumab in patients with pretreated advanced melanoma. Journal of Clinical Oncology. 2016;**34**:1330-1338. DOI: 10.1200/JCO.2015.63.4121

[49] Spanggaard I, Snoj M, Cavalcanti A, et al. Gene electrotransfer of plasmid antiangiogenic metargidin peptide (AMEP) in disseminated melanoma: Safety and efficacy results of a phase I first-in-man study. Human Gene Therapy Clinical Development. 2013;**24**:99-107. DOI: 10.1089/humc.2012.240

[50] Daud AI, DeConti RC, Andrews S, et al. Phase I trial of interleukin-12 plasmid electroporation in patients with metastatic melanoma. Journal of Clinical Oncology. 2008;**26**:5896-5903. DOI: 10.1200/JCO.2007.15.6794

[51] Spanggaard I, Dahlstroem K, Laessoee L, et al. Gene therapy for patients with advanced solid tumors: A phase I study using gene electrotransfer to muscle with the integrin inhibitor plasmid AMEP. Acta Oncologica (Madr). 2017;**56**:909-916. DOI: 10.1080/0284186X.2017.1315171

[52] Liu F, Song Y, Liu D. Hydrodynamics-based transfection in animals by systemic administration of plasmid DNA. Gene Therapy. 1999;**6**:1258-1266. DOI: 10.1038/sj.gt.3300947

[53] Zhang G, Budker V, Wolff JA. High levels of foreign gene expression in hepatocytes after tail vein injections of naked plasmid DNA. Human Gene Therapy. 1999;**10**:1735-1737. DOI: 10.1089/10430349950017734

[54] Suda T, Suda K, Liu D. Computer-assisted hydrodynamic gene delivery. Molecular Therapy. 2008;**16**:1098-1104. DOI: 10.1038/mt.2008.66

[55] Kamimura K, Zhang G, Liu D. Image-guided, intravascular hydrodynamic gene delivery to skeletal muscle in pigs. Molecular Therapy. 2010;**18**:93-100. DOI: 10.1038/mt.2009.206

[56] Kamimura K, Suda T, Xu W, et al. Image-guided, lobe-specific hydrodynamic gene delivery to swine liver. Molecular Therapy. 2009;**17**:491-499. DOI: 10.1038/mt.2008.294

[57] Sendra L, Pérez D, Miguel A, et al. Human AAT gene transfer to pig liver improved by using a perfusion isolated organ endovascular procedure. European Radiology. 2016;**26**: 95-102. DOI: 10.1007/s00330-015-3792-2

[58] Yokoo T, Kamimura K, Abe H, et al. Liver-targeted hydrodynamic gene therapy: Recent advances in the technique. World Journal of Gastroenterology. 2016;**22**:8862. DOI: 10.3748/wjg.v22.i40.8862

[59] Kamimura K, Kanefuji T, Yokoo T, et al. Safety assessment of liver-targeted hydrodynamic gene delivery in dogs. PLoS One. 2014;**9**:e107203. DOI: 10.1371/journal.pone.0107203

[60] Wooddell CI, Hegge JO, Zhang G, et al. Dose response in rodents and nonhuman primates after hydrodynamic limb vein delivery of naked plasmid DNA. Human Gene Therapy. 2011;**22**:889-903. DOI: 10.1089/hum.2010.160

[61] Hagstrom JE, Hegge J, Zhang G, et al. A facile nonviral method for delivering genes and siRNAs to skeletal muscle of mammalian limbs. Molecular Therapy. 2004;**10**:386-398. DOI: 10.1016/j.ymthe.2004.05.004

[62] Anavi S, Hahn-Obercyger M, Margalit R, et al. A novel antihypoglycemic role of inducible nitric oxide synthase in liver inflammatory response induced by dietary cholesterol and endotoxemia. Antioxidants & Redox Signaling. 2013;**19**:1889-1901. DOI: 10.1089/ars.2012.5157

[63] McCaffrey AP, Meuse L, Pham T-TT, et al. RNA interference in adult mice. Nature. 2002; **418**:38-39. DOI: 10.1038/418038a

[64] Bonamassa B, Hai L, Liu D. Hydrodynamic gene delivery and its applications in pharmaceutical research. Pharmaceutical Research. 2011;**28**:694-701. DOI: 10.1007/s11095-010-0338-9

[65] Huang M, Sun R, Wei H, et al. Simultaneous knockdown of multiple ligands of innate receptor NKG2D prevents natural killer cell-mediated fulminant hepatitis in mice. Hepatology. 2013;**57**:277-288. DOI: 10.1002/hep.25959

[66] Chen S-W, Zhang X-R, Wang C-Z, et al. RNA interference targeting the platelet-derived growth factor receptor beta subunit ameliorates experimental hepatic fibrosis in rats. Liver International. 2008;**28**:1446-1457. DOI: 10.1111/j.1478-3231.2008.01759.x

[67] Abe H, Kamimura K, Kobayashi Y, et al. Effective prevention of liver fibrosis by liver-targeted hydrodynamic gene delivery of matrix metalloproteinase-13 in a rat liver fibrosis model. Molecular Therapy–Nucleic Acids. 2016;**5**:e276. DOI: 10.1038/mtna.2015.49

[68] Tsai S, Wang W. Expression and function of fibroblast growth factor (FGF) 7 during liver regeneration. Cellular Physiology and Biochemistry. 2011;**27**:641-652

[69] Ochoa MC, Fioravanti J, Duitman EH, et al. Liver gene transfer of interkeukin-15 constructs that become part of circulating high density lipoproteins for immunotherapy. PLoS One. 2012;**7**:e52370. Epub ahead of print. DOI: 10.1371/journal.pone.0052370

[70] Suda T, Gao X, Stolz DB, et al. Structural impact of hydrodynamic injection on mouse liver. Gene Therapy. 2007;**14**:129-137. DOI: 10.1038/sj.gt.3302865

[71] Kanefuji T, Yokoo T, Suda T, et al. Hemodynamics of a hydrodynamic injection. Molecular Therapy–Methods & Clinical Development. 2014;**1**:14029. DOI: 10.1038/mtm.2014.29

[72] Miao CH, Ye X, Thompson AR. High-level factor VIII gene expression in vivo achieved by nonviral liver-specific gene therapy vectors. Human Gene Therapy. 2003;**14**:1297-1305. DOI: 10.1089/104303403322319381

[73] Zender L, Hutker S, Liedtke C, et al. Caspase 8 small interfering RNA prevents acute liver failure in mice. Proceedings of the National Academy of Sciences of the United States of America. 2003;**100**:7797-7802. DOI: 10.1073/pnas.1330920100

[74] Shigekawa M, Hikita H, Kodama T, et al. Pancreatic STAT3 protects mice against caerulein-induced pancreatitis via PAP1 induction. The American Journal of Pathology. 2012;**181**:2105-2113. DOI: 10.1016/j.ajpath.2012.08.038

[75] Maruyama H, Higuchi N, Nishikawa Y, et al. Kidney-targeted naked DNA transfer by retrograde renal vein injection in rats. Human Gene Therapy. 2002;**13**:455-468. DOI: 10.1089/10430340252792585

[76] Ogawa K, Kamimura K, Kobayashi Y, et al. Efficacy and safety of pancreas-targeted hydrodynamic gene delivery in rats. Molecular Therapy–Nucleic Acids. 2017;**9**:80-88. DOI: 10.1016/j.omtn.2017.08.009

[77] Yokoo T, Kamimura K, Suda T, et al. Novel electric power-driven hydrodynamic injection system for gene delivery: Safety and efficacy of human factor IX delivery in rats. Gene Therapy. 2013;**20**:816-823. DOI: 10.1038/gt.2013.2

[78] Kamimura K, Suda T, Zhang G, et al. Parameters affecting image-guided, hydrodynamic gene delivery to swine liver. Molecular Therapy–Nucleic Acids. 2013;**2**:e128. DOI: 10.1038/mtna.2013.52

[79] Yokoo T, Kanefuji T, Suda T, et al. Site-specific impact of a regional hydrodynamic injection: Computed tomography study during hydrodynamic injection targeting the swine liver. Pharmaceutics. 2015;7:334-343. DOI: 10.3390/pharmaceutics7030334

Chapter 2

Gene Therapy for Cystic Fibrosis: Hurdles to Overcome for Successful Clinical Translation

Myriam Sainz-Ramos, Nuseibah AL Qtaish,
Idoia Gallego, Ilia Villate-Beitia, Tania López,
Gustavo Puras and José Luis Pedraz

Additional information is available at the end of the chapter

http://dx.doi.org/10.5772/intechopen.79719

Abstract

Cystic fibrosis (CF) is a genetic disease that hampers the lung function. Despite that the main defective gene has been deeply characterized, some relevant concerns still need to be resolved before considering gene therapy as a realistic medical choice. One of the major issues that need to be strongly considered in order to succeed in the search for an effective gene therapy approach for CF is the design of the appropriate genetic material to be delivered. Other relevant factors to take into consideration include the design of safe and effective gene delivery systems, the biological barriers that need to be overcome in order to reach the nucleus of the target cells, and the problems related to the design of a drug formulation suitable for lung delivery purposes. Furthermore, some problems related to the commercialization of gene therapy products also need to be resolved. In this chapter, we discuss the up-to-date strategies to overcome such hurdles in order for gene therapy to become a routine treatment modality for CF.

Keywords: cystic fibrosis, gene therapy, drug delivery, biological barriers, drug formulation

1. Introduction

Cystic fibrosis (CF) is a rare disease with low prevalence caused by the dysfunction of the transmembrane conductance regulatory gene (CFTR). The most prevalent CFTR mutation consists of a deletion of a phenylalanine at position 508 [1]. The disease presents a heterogeneous distribution in the world population being more frequent in Northern Europe.

According to recent reports, in the European Union, 1 of every 2000–3000 newborns is affected by CF. In the USA, the incidence is 1 per 3500 births. In Asia, the predisposition to CF is low; however, there is evidence to show that this disease is severely underdiagnosed [2]. The basic characteristic of CF is the transport of defective ions in the apical membrane of most secretory cells, which leads to an altered secretion of mucus in the epithelium of the respiratory tract, the digestive tract, the pancreas, the liver, and the reproductive track [1]. The conventional treatments available on market, which include, among others, antibiotics, pancreatic enzyme supplements, high-fat diets, and even physiotherapy [3], afford the consequences derived from CFTR dysfunction and have significantly improved the mean life expectancy of patients affected by the disease up to 34 years [4]. However, their quality of life is severely compromised mainly due to side effects and interactions among such treatments [5]. Therefore, other therapeutic options such as gene therapy, in which the main goal is to restore the function of the mutated CFTR protein acting on the genetic cause of the problem, need to be considered. CFTR gene was cloned more than two decades ago, and the monogenic and autosomal recessive nature of CF disease means that the addition and expression of the corrected gene could reverse the underlying cause of the disease. Therefore, there is reasonable hope to consider gene therapy as a potential realistic medical option, and consequently, some clinical trials have been performed since 1993. However, despite the moderate optimism that emerged with the development of such clinical assays, there are still some hurdles to overcome before considering gene therapy a realistic medical option. Main concerns are related to the intrinsic properties of genetic materials, the development of safe and efficient gene delivery vectors able to deliver genetic materials to the nucleus of target cells, the design of a drug formulation suitable for pulmonary gene delivery applications, and the hurdles associated with the commercialization of such drugs (**Figure 1**).

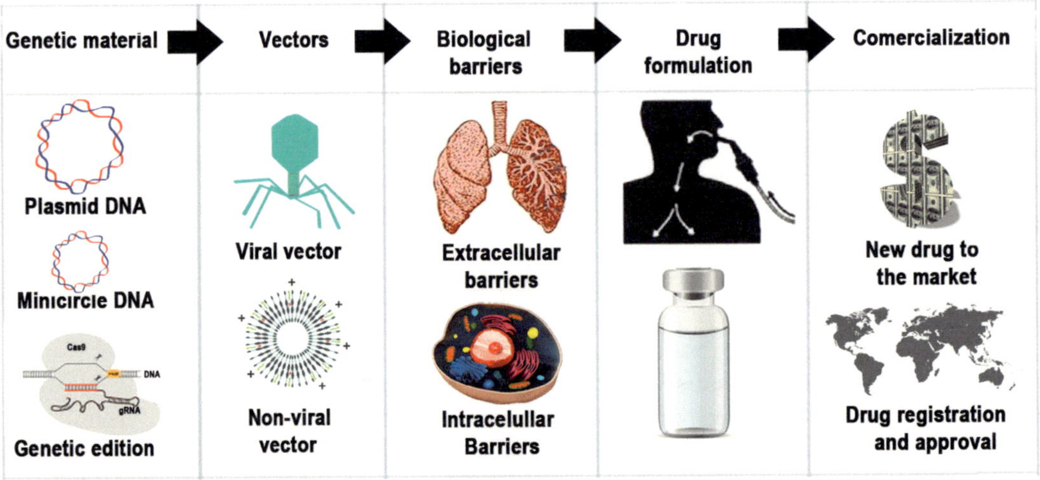

Figure 1. Hurdles that gene therapy should overcome in order to reach clinical practice in the treatment of CF disease.

In the next sections, we will analyze such barriers along with the most relevant approaches developed by the scientific community to circumvent them in order to cure CF with gene therapy.

2. Genetic material

2.1. Plasmid DNA

Bacterial plasmid DNA (pDNA) remains an interesting biomolecule for gene transfer, with several promising reports and clinical trials in progress worldwide [6]. In CF, pDNA has been successfully delivered by nonviral vectors to the sheep lung [7]. Additionally, when administered in multiple-dosage regimen, no loss of activity was observed [8]. In order to be produced in recombinant bacteria and to express their therapeutic gene of interest (GOI), pDNA needs a bacterial origin of replication sequence (bac-ORI). In addition, pDNA backbone includes a sequence with resistance to one/various antibiotics such as kanamycin, which allows to select the clone of bacteria transformed that expresses the plasmid. Finally, a eukaryotic promoter is needed to enhance GOI expression [9]. Usually, when pDNA reaches the nucleus of target cells, it remains in an episomal position, which means that it replicates independently from the host chromosomal DNA, avoiding the undesirable activation of oncogenic genes [10]. The main concerns of pDNA in gene therapy are related to safety issues. Classically, in eukaryotic cells, pDNA has been associated with the induction of undesired immune responses and secretion of proinflammatory cytokines [11]. For instance, a transient neutrophilic infiltration and an elevation in proinflammatory cytokines have been reported in mouse lung [12]. Although the episomal nature of pDNA could be an interesting advantage, the transfection efficiency remains compromised mainly by the transient and relatively low gene expression. Additionally, the size of the plasmid, determined by the number of base pairs, jeopardizes transfection efficiency [13, 14].

2.2. Minicircle DNA

In order to overcome the previously mentioned disadvantages associated with the use of pDNA in gene therapy, small plasmidic cassettes known as minicircle DNAs (mcDNAs) have been recently developed [15]. Cameron and Scheleff first employed mcDNA terminology in 1995. Nowadays, this technology offers a potential alternative to enhance both transfection efficiency and safety of gene delivery [14]. Basically, mcDNAs are circular constructors similar to pDNA but significantly smaller, since mcDNAs contain a minimal expression cassette, of a promoter, a transgene, and a polyadenylation, signal but are devoid of bacterial pDNA elements. Thus, mcDNA technology allows sustained transgene expression mainly due to a lower activation of nuclear transgene silencing mechanisms and reduced immunogenic responses in vivo [16, 17].

In the lung, some promising results have been obtained with the use of small plasmidic cassettes [18]. In fact, results of a Phase IIb double-blind clinical trial for CF have been recently reported. These trials were performed with a plasmid encoding CFTR gene and lacking CpG bacterial region, known as pGM169 [8]. In such study, treated patients exhibited modest but significant improvements in lung function compared to placebo-treated ones during 1-year follow-up [19]. In any case, despite the optimism generated, there are still some concerns that need to be considered, such as the reproducibility of the results; the intensity of the response, probably conditioned by the degradation of formulation after aerosolization process; or the number of patients that received such treatment.

2.3. Genome editing tools

Both previously mentioned approaches based on pDNA and mcDNA technologies allow to restore the function of the mutated CFTR gene, with the addition of normal copies, but they do not correct the mutation at their local chromosomal location. However, genome editing tools based on zinc-finger nucleases (ZFNs), or transcription activator-like effector nucleases (TALENs), can specifically correct CFTR gene mutations at their natural chromosomal location, and so, the corrected gene can remain under the control of its endogenous promoter [20].

ZFNs are synthetic restriction enzymes, which have three or more zinc-finger DNA-binding motifs linked to the FokI restriction enzyme that recognizes trinucleotides in a specific DNA sequence [21]. When FokI enzyme creates a double-strand break (DSB) near the mutation place, cellular DNA repair mechanisms are activated to maintain cell viability. In these conditions, a donor DNA sequence with high 5′ and 3′ homology with the DNA sequence where DSB has been generated can be exogenously supplemented to enhance the correction of the mutation by homologous recombination (HR) mechanism. This genome editing tool has been successfully used in vitro to correct CFTRΔF508 mutation in both human bronchial epithelial cells [22] and CF-induced pluripotent stem (IPS) cells [23].

TALEN technology is very similar to ZFNs. These nucleases were originally characterized in *Xanthomonas* bacteria, in which TALEN proteins are secreted when *Xanthomonas* infect a wide variety of plants, thus activating genes that help to develop the pathogenesis. This genome editing tool also produces a DSB around the mutation site of the target gene and consequently induces cellular DNA repair mechanisms [24]. TALENs are considered as a more efficient and cost-effective alternative to ZFNs [25]. In the case of ZFNs, each finger module recognizes three to four bases of the DNA sequence. However, in the case of TALENs, gene recognition is mediated by a more specific mechanism, where each module of 33–35 amino acid targets a single nucleotide. This technology has been recently applied to correct CFTRΔF508 mutations in CF patient-specific IPS cells [26]. Overall, such study reported correction of patient-specific IPS cells in less than 3 months, which could allow rapid scaling up for future applications.

Clustered regularly interspaced short palindromic repeats (CRISPR) methodology, originally described as an adaptive immune response in archaea, follows the same rationale described for ZFNs and TALENs, but instead of protein domains, short RNA molecules are used to drive the required homology [27]. In this case, an endonuclease called Cas9 is guided by a single guide RNA (gRNA) to hybridize specifically with the mutated sequence in the DNA; then, as described for ZFNs and TALENs, the resulting DSB triggers cellular DNA repair mechanism [28]. The main advantage of CRISPR technology is that it is an easy-to-synthesize cost-effective tool that is able to correct more than one mutation at the same time, if multiple-gene targeted sgRNAs are delivered to target cell along with the Cas9 protein, which makes it an excellent option [24]. CRISPR technology has been applied to repair CFTRΔF508 mutations in intestinal stem cell organoids of CF patients [29].

This study represents an interesting proof of concept for CFTRΔF508 correction by HR using CRISPR/Cas9 technology in primary adult stem cells derived from patients with a single-gene hereditary defect and offers reasonable hope to be successfully applied to the lungs of patients affected by CF. However, some relevant concerns, mainly related to the frequency of undesirable off targets, still need to be resolved in order to reach clinical practice [19].

3. Vectors

One of the main concerns related to the clinical application of gene therapy is the design and development of safe and effective gene delivery vectors to introduce exogenous genetic material into the nucleus of target cells [30, 31]. In the absence of gene delivery vectors, naked genetic material is quickly degraded mainly by exogenous deoxyribonuclease enzymes, which clearly inhibit transfection efficiency [31]. Additionally, the negatively charged genetic material, mainly due to the phosphate groups, hampers the electrostatic interactions with cell membranes, which are negatively charged too. Therefore, the clinical application of gene therapy demands the design, characterization, and evaluation of efficient and safe carriers to mammalian cells.

3.1. Viral vectors

At present, viral-based carriers are the most appropriate from an effectiveness point of view. The natural evolution that viruses have undergone over many years has allowed them to face different intra- and extracellular barriers and, consequently, infect target cells with high efficiency.

In the CF field, a wide variety of viral-based vectors has been developed in clinical trials. The first one was performed in 1993 with adenovirus in three patients, where partial correction of the chloride transport in nasal epithelium was observed [32]. Some of the main advantages of adenoviruses include their non integrating nature and their natural tropism for the lung. However, despite such favorable properties, and the high transduction efficiency observed in most tissues, gene expression usually remains transient, and these viruses can induce strong immune and inflammatory responses in a dose-dependent manner, which clearly brings up safety issues and, therefore, limits their application in the clinical practice [8].

Initial clinical trials performed with adenovirus allowed the development of adeno-associated viruses (AAV), which have interesting characteristics for their application in gene therapy, such as broad tissue tropism, high transduction efficieny, and persistent episomal expression, which can last for years, even though it is a non integrating vector [33, 34]. In addition, recombinant AAV vectors have been shown to be safe in several clinical trials, as they are not related to any known human disease. However, these vectors also present relevant limitations, the main one being their low capacity to load genetic material (<5 kb) [35]. Between

1999 and 2007, six clinical trials were conducted with these kinds of vectors in CF [8]. Phase I clinical trials demonstrated that a single-dose administration of AAV in the respiratory tract of patients affected by CF was safe and well tolerated [36]. Nevertheless, subsequent studies, with repeated doses in more patients, did not report significant improvement in lung function [37]. This lack of efficacy was mainly attributed to the low DNA loading capacity of AAV, which prevented loading the 4.7 kb of the CFTR gene [8]. In addition, AAV capsid-specific immune responses limited repeated administrations in patients [8]. Nowadays, some interesting strategies are being developed in order to minimize adaptive immune responses after repeated administration, such as the design of hybrid AAV capsids or the removal of CpG bacterial regions from AAV vectors [38, 39].

Lentiviruses have an integrative nature and have shown long-term and stable transgene expression when administered in the respiratory tract of mice, which minimizes the need for repeated administration [40]. Additionally, the packaging of full-length CFTR gene and promoters is not limited by size. Therefore, nowadays they are considered promising vectors for the treatment of CF [41]. However, in order to consider its use in clinical practice, some concerns still need to be resolved, such as the scaling in the production of these vectors and the control of the place where the transgene is inserted into the genome of the pulmonary cells, which could increase the tumorigenicity potential of such viral vectors due to random integration [20]. Consequently, such viral vectors could be more suitable for ex vivo than for in vivo therapy. In any case, a promising study in three newborn CF pigs has recently shown that 2 weeks after lentiviral delivery by aerosolization, the anion channel defect can be corrected in a large animal CF model [42]. Other recent studies assessed with pseudotyped lentivirus vectors in both murine lungs and human air-liquid interface cultures showed that preexisting and acquired immune responses do not interfere with vector efficacy [43]. In such study, at least 14% of the airway cells were transduced. Interestingly, toxicological results, notably the integration site profile showing absence of integration near oncogenic loci, support further progression toward clinical trials.

3.2. Nonviral vectors

Although the use of viral-based vectors in clinical trials still predominates over that of nonviral vectors, in recent years, there has been a notable increase in preclinical studies using nonviral vectors [44]. The reason is that these systems represent a safer, cheaper, and easier to produce alternative to viral-based vectors [18]. The main advantages of nonviral vectors include, among others, the ability to produce them on a large scale with high reproducibility and low cost; their relative stability after storage; the possibility of multiple-dose regimen administration due to their low immunogenicity; their high capacity to carry genetic material, independently of the size [45]; as well as the possibility to modify them chemically in order to regulate important physicochemical parameters, such as size, charge, morphology, or polydispersion, which clearly influence their final biological properties. All these important advantages have raised the interest of the scientific community to develop new biocompatible materials of different structures, compositions, sizes, and characteristics to transport therapeutic genes into specific organs or cells, overcoming the different extra- and intracellular barriers [46].

Within the large variety of nonviral vectors developed, most of them are based on peptides as well as on cationic lipids and polymers, which form the corresponding complexes (polyplexes and lipoplexes) after electrostatic binding with DNA [47]. The resulting complexes protect nucleic acids from enzymatic degradation and facilitate cellular uptake by interactions with the cytoplasmic membrane [48]. The PEG-CK30 peptide, due to its low immunogenicity and its ability to be endocytosed by cells, is one of the most widely used, although the formulation must be optimized to allow its administration in aerosol form to reach the lungs [49].

Regarding cationic polymers, polyethylenimine (PEI) is one of the most used, since its chemical structure can be easily modified to increase the efficiency of transfection, for example, by incorporating lactose (Lac-PEI) to improve intracellular trafficking [50]. However, PEI has not yet been used in any clinical trial. The main limitation lies in the difficulty that exists to prepare PEI polyplexes at high DNA concentrations [49]. One of the most promising strategies that have been used to circumvent this problem is the use of ultrafiltration methods, through which PEI/DNA concentrates are prepared.

In the case of cationic lipids, some of the most widely used to develop nonviral formulations in the CF field are N-[1-(2,3-dioleyloxy) propyl]-N, N, N-trimethylammonium, dioleoylphosphatidyl ethanolamine, and dioleoyl trimethyl ammonium [51]. However, currently, the most promising nonviral vector in CF clinical trials is based on the cationic lipid GL6TA, which was synthesized to prevent DNA degradation in the lysosome and to be stable after pulmonary administration by aerosolization [8, 51]. In 2011, a preclinical comparative study of the use of PEI, PEG-CK30, or GL67A nonviral vectors in aerosols demonstrated that this last formulation was the best one to transport DNA to sheep's lungs [7]. Moreover, in an extensive preclinical study performed in 2014 [52], it was corroborated that the formulation based on the lipid GL67A, which had already been used for 15 years in CF clinical trials, was still suitable for administration in multiple-dose regimen, without any observed loss of activity [8].

4. Biological barriers

In order to reach the nucleus of target cells and initiate transgene expression, the genetic material must overcome some extracellular and intracellular barriers, which will be discussed in this section, along with the most relevant strategies that have been developed to make the transfection process more efficient.

4.1. Extracellular barriers

Even though intravenous injection is one of the most commonly used administration routes, especially for delivering genetic cargo into cancerous cells, some barriers still hamper its use in clinical practice, particularly in the CF disease [53]. First of all, the genetic material needs to be protected against extracellular enzymatic digestion, since DNA is quickly degraded when administered alone. To avoid such quick degradation, nonviral vectors based on both positively charged lipids and polymers offer the possibility to condense on their surface the genetic material by electrostatic interactions and minimize such undesirable effect [54].

However, the final positive charge of polyplexes or lipoplexes can interact in a nonspecific way, not only with target cell membranes but also with other negatively charged components such as serum proteins that jeopardize transfection efficiency [55]. These interactions could result in the formation of aggregates that classically are eliminated from the blood by the reticuloendothelial system. Interestingly, the incorporation of polyethylene glycol (PEG) motifs into the formulation of some nonviral carriers enhances the stability of complexes, since the highly hydrophobic nature of PEG chains creates a steric barrier to prevent both aggregation of complexes in blood circulation and extracellular enzymatic degradation by nucleases [55]. In any case, other relevant aspects related with both the length and the degree of PEGylation should be also considered, as they can also decrease DNA condensation efficiency with nanoparticles [56]. In addition to PEG, other polymers with hydrophobic nature such as poly(4-acryloylmorpholine) or poly(N,N-dimethylacrylamide) have recently emerged as interesting and promising alternatives to compensate or ameliorate the negative effects associated with PEGylation [57].

Since intravenous injections present relevant hurdles that hamper the delivery of genetic material into target lung cells, local administration into the lung seems to be a reasonable alternative. In this case, the presence of mucus and the clearance mechanism are the most relevant barriers to overcome [58]. To avoid such barriers associated with pulmonary administration, other interesting noninvasive routes of administration, such as intranasal instillation, can be used to target lung cells. Nevertheless, the main problem is the low amount of genetic material that can be administered by the intranasal route. From a technical point of view, aerosolized nonviral vector/DNA complexes, carefully designed for inhalation in combination with appropriate excipients to enhance both particle flow and aerodynamic diameter, could be an interesting option since they are needle-free systems able to deliver locally high cargo concentrations [53].

To circumvent the diffusion of complexes into lung cells due to unspecific interactions with the biopolymer network of the mucus, some mucolytic agents that hydrolyze mucins can be added [58]. Other strategies include the incorporation of N-acetylcysteine to reduce disulfide bridges between the subunits of mucin, and consequently the viscosity [59], or the functionalization of nonviral vector formulations with mucolytic agents.

4.2. Intracellular barriers

Once extracellular barriers are overcome, there is still a long way full of hurdles before reaching the nucleus of target cells. Firstly, complexes carrying the genetic material need to be endocytosed by target cells. The interaction between complexes and cell membranes can occur in an unspecific way or can be mediated by a specific ligand, which is the preferred one, especially for in vivo applications [60]. Of note, the choice of ligand to be incorporated into the nanoparticle formulation depends not only on the target cell but also on the type of cell entry pathway that will be used once the ligand binds to the desired receptor.

Classically, there are four main pathways of endocytosis: clathrin-mediated endocytosis (CME), caveolae-mediated endocytosis (CVME), phagocytosis, and macropinocytosis [61, 62]. CME is an energy-dependent mechanism widely studied and characterized [63]. Typically, this pathway is directly associated with lysosomes, where the genetic material needs to leave such biological compartment quickly before being degraded by the acidic environment and the enzymes found in lysosomes [63]. To avoid this enzymatic degradation, some interesting strategies can be used, such as the formation of pores in the endosome membrane by incorporation of amphiphilic cationic peptides. This creates strong internal tensions in the membrane and enhances the exit of endosome content through such pores [64]. Another strategy is known as the "proton sponge effect," where the low pH within the endosome allows the protonation of trapped compounds that have a large capacity to absorb protons from the medium (buffer effect). Such protonation causes an important entry of ions (H^+ and Cl^-) and water in the endosome, which produce a swelling effect and its rupture. This effect has been observed in some cationic polymers with high buffering capacity over a wide pH range [64]. In CVME, internalized molecules go to the caveosome instead of lysosome [61] avoiding lysosomal degradation; however, there is still ongoing debate, with some authors claiming that CVME can fuse with lysosomes [65].

Phagocytosis is a special type of endocytosis used mainly by macrophages, monocytes, neutrophils, and dendritic cells, although other cell types can also use this cellular entry pathway [61]. Endocytosis mediated by phagocytosis comprises the formation of membrane extensions with certain forms to capture particles generally greater than 1 μm. In contrast, for endocytosis mediated by macropinocytosis, membrane extensions do not surround particles but form some kind of protuberances that finally fuse with the cytoplasmic membrane. In many cases, the physicochemical properties of nonviral vector-based nanoparticles, such as particle size, superficial charge, morphology, or polydispersity, directly influence the endocytosis mechanism and consequently the transfection efficiency.

Once the DNA is released into the cytosol of cells, it must enter the nucleus to produce its effect. This is considered a significant barrier that nonviral vectors must overcome in order to mediate a good transfection efficiency. One commonly used strategy to enhance nuclear import of genetic material is to incorporate a nuclear localization signal (NLS), such as polylysine or protamine [66]. NLS contains some amino acids that interact with some proteins of the cytoplasm known as importines. These importins enhance nuclear entry through the nuclear pore complex of the nuclear membrane through an energy-dependent mechanism [67].

5. Drug formulation

The airways seem to be the natural way to treat respiratory diseases and a good alternative to systemic and more invasive procedures. Currently, aerosolization is the prefered method of administration for airway targeting since it is a noninvasive route that induces little stress to patients. Moreover, high quantities of drug can be deposited directly and fast into the lungs, which circumvents the blood circulation and avoids the first-pass effect of the liver. However, the effectiveness of such approach strongly depends on the development of smart drug formulation strategies. One of the critical steps that need to be taken into account for a successful gene delivery approach by inhalation is the formulation of the drug molecules into an appropriate inhalable form with sufficient stability and adequate aerodynamic properties [68]. Highly susceptible molecules, such as nucleic acid, require special attention when delivered by this route of administration. The physicochemical constraints such as the hydrodynamic shear forces generated during aerosolization can induce degradation of the nucleic acids, which will be more or less important depending on their size [69, 70]. Therefore, the need to develop a suitable formulation able to protect the material from degradation and at the same time ensure delivery of nucleic acid to the target cells in the lung needs to be deeply considered. In this sense, the commonly accepted aerodynamic size for pulmonary gene delivery is within the range of 1–5 μm. Larger particles (4–7 μm) tend to deposit in the airways, while smaller particles (1–3 μm) and those in submicron range (<1 μm) reach the lower airways and deeper lung [68]. The aerodynamic diameter of a particle can be modified not only by changing its size but also by varying its density or shape, which opens new possible strategies for gene delivery to the lung, such as the design of large porous hollow particles [71].

Suitable formulations for pulmonary delivery are mainly prepared either by dissolving or by suspending the therapeutic molecules in a liquid or formulating them into a dry powder for inhalation using liquid inhalers (including nebulizers), dry powder inhalers (DPIs), or pressurized metered dose inhalers (pMDIs); each of them is suitable for different applications. Once the aerosolized droplets or microparticles are deposited next to the target location into the lungs, they need to dissolve in the lung lining fluid for subsequent absorption and cellular uptake [72]. Nowadays, viral gene delivery to the lungs is limited to liquid formulations using a nebulizer [36], and there is no dry powder or metered dose inhaler formulation available for any vector-drug combination. In most cases, the gene transfer efficiency to lung cells using viral vectors is still too low with traditional nebulizer devices, probably due to the degradation of viral envelope by the shear forces caused during aerosolization [73] and the viscous mucus found in obstructive diseases, like CF [74]. Moreover, and as previously highlighted, the use of adenoviral or AAV vectors would likely induce an acute immune response upon the initial administration or result in low efficacy following repeat dosing. This is particularly relevant since aerosolized gene therapy might require repeat dosing because mucus clearance mechanisms and/or phagocytes may engulf and destroy the drug vector before it can be taken up by target cells [75]. In contrast, the simpler composition of nonviral vectors may have, in this case, an advantage over viral vectors, making readministration potentially more successful.

Although pulmonary gene-based therapies have not yet been granted marketing approval, numerous strategies are being tested both in vitro and in vivo, and various clinical trials are underway [19, 36]. **Table 1** summarizes some of the strategies used to date for the pulmonary delivery of nucleic acids by aerosolization.

Nowadays, the most studied approach for gene delivery to the lung involves the nebulization of the selected formulation [76], turning it from a liquid solution to microdroplets. Depending on the aerosolization system used, such as jet, ultrasonic, or mesh nebulizers, the implemented hydrodynamic stress that the therapeutic molecules would be subject to varies [77]. Interestingly, several strategies have been studied to reduce the damage to the genetic material during the aerosolization process, by condensing the nucleic acids with positively charged molecules, such as polyethylenimine (PEI), protamine, or poly-L-lysine (PLL), among others [78].

Description	Vector	Aerosolization	References
In vivo aerosol delivery of PEI-DNA comp	PEI	Nebulization	[68]
Randomized, double-blind, placebo-controlled, Phase II trial in CF patients with mild lung disease	AAV2 viral	Nebulization	[32]
Nebulization of receptor-targeted nanocomplexes for in vivo gene delivery to the airway epithelium	Receptor-targeting peptides and cationic liposomes	Nebulization	[69]
In vivo repeated aerosol delivery of pDNA/PEI complexes with CpG-free plasmids	PEI	Nebulization or instillation	[70]
In vivo aerosol delivery of DNA/liposomes to the lung	GL67A cationic liposomes	Multiple nebulizers	[71]
Randomized, double-blind, placebo-controlled, Phase IIb trial	GL67A cationic liposomes	Nebulization	[14]
In vivo intratracheal administration of pDNA-chitosan dry powders, obtained by SFD	Chitosan	Dry powder, obtained by SFD, administered by intratracheal syringe	[72]
Dry powder aerosols for in vivo gene delivery to the lung	PEI	Dry powder in insufflator lyophilization/powderization with lactose, sucrose, or trehalose	[73]

Table 1. Pulmonary gene delivery strategies by aerosolization.

The elaboration of DPIs, composed of drug-based dry powders and an aerosol-generating device, also presents important advantages such as high physicochemical stability, easy handling, and propellant-free aerosols. In order to transform the therapeutic nucleic acids into stable dry powders, several techniques, such as freeze-drying (FD) [79], spray-drying (SD) [80], and spray freeze-drying (SFD) [81], are being investigated. In addition, the incorporation of suitable stabilizing agents/thermal protectors such as polysaccharides (sucrose [79], trehalose [79], agarose [82], lactose [83], mannitol [81], or chitosan [84]), amino acids (leucine [84] or glycine [82]), or proteins (BSA [85]) is critical.

6. Commercialization

In addition to the above concerns, other relevant issues specifically related to the commercialization of gene therapy medicinal products (GTMP) must also be considered. Commercially available medical products based on gene therapy along with cell therapy and tissue engineering are classified as advanced therapy medicinal products. Although highly promising, their translation into clinical practice is nowadays hampered by major critical issues such as complex regulatory and ethical aspects, along with the intrinsic difficulties to scale up these products to an industrial level [20].

Regarding the regulatory concerns of GTMP that affect clinical applications, the economical investments, along with their manufacture and control, demand more attention than chemically synthesized small molecules [86]. Therefore, a deep analysis of both costs and benefits needs to be done before considering the commercialization of such therapies [87].

Another relevant concern that jeopardizes the clinical use of GTMP in CF is the ethical aspect of clinical trials. Since the early 1990s, more than 25 Phase I gene therapy clinical trials have been conducted. These trials have been carried out largely to assess the safety and feasibility of gene transfer methods and their expression in the host, reporting variable successes for both viral and nonviral approaches. Gene therapy products designed for the treatment of CF must meet certain requirements in order to become a viable therapeutic option. For instance, their clinical efficacy must be demonstrated by analyzing appropriate variables of the lung function such as the patient´s vital capacity that they are able to expire in the first second of forced expiration (FEV1), their age, sex or body composition, and the therapeutic efficacy which must be maintained with repeated administrations. In addition, the GTMP must demonstrate an acceptable profile when it comes to side effects, and other considerations such as treatment of early versus established lung disease must also be analysed.

Since a high percentage of patients affected by CF are children, clinical trials involving these patients must carefully balance the potential benefits of these therapies and the associated risks [88]. Regarding this controversial issue, the Gene Therapy Advisory Committee recommends that clinical trials on children should only be performed under specific circumstances, whereby: (i) it has been demonstrated that the research is necessary to promote the health of the trial population, (ii) the research cannot be done in adults, and (iii) there is a high potential of therapeutic benefit [88]. In fact, owing to a demonstrated benefit of early gene therapy intervention, the age of enrolment of children in clinical trials has progressively reduced over the years from 18 to 12 years old. However, parents should have legal rights to make the final decision on behalf of their children.

Another critical hurdle that strongly compromises the clinical application of gene therapy products for the treatment of CF is the difficulty to scale up formulations that were originally developed for basic clinical research [89]. Most of these products are usually developed by small- and medium-sized enterprises, in collaboration with academic groups, which are usually highly engaged in preclinical activities, but have limited manufacturing experience at industrial level. For instance, the normal procedure for preparing nonviral-based gene therapy products is by simply mixing and pipetting the negatively charged genetic material and the positively charged polymer - or lipid-based nonviral vector formulations, which are often produced in the laboratory at small volumes that usually oscillate between 1 and 5 mL. However, the standardization of this procedure at industrial level to produce high and stable levels of complexes under GMP conditions represents a great challenge that needs to be overcome for successful clinical application. In this sense, pilot plants, which employ small volumes of the product, represent an interesting option to gain knowledge on the technical process before full scale up production.

7. Conclusion

Despite the fact that the CFTR gene was cloned two decades ago, the current, conventional treatments for CF focus on masking the main symptoms, rather than addressing the underlying genetic cause of the disease. In this sense, gene therapy represents a promising alternative to tackle CF, considering the autosomal recessive nature of the most relevant ΔF508 mutation. Although the main objective of gene therapy seems simple, there are some hurdles that need to be overcome before gene therapy for CF becomes a realistic treatment option. In any case, the increase in knowledge and recent advances in biopharmaceutical technology offer reasonable hope for the treatment of this devastating disease. The minicircle technology, along with the new gene editing tools, offer important advantages compared with classical plasmids used to add functional copies of the gene. Additionally, intense research in novel nonviral vectors functionalized to overcome both extra- and intracellular barriers and the possibility to aerosolize such formulations without losing activity merit special attention.

Acknowledgements

This project was supported by the Basque Country Government (Department of Education, University and Research, predoctoral grant PRE_2016_2_0302 and Consolidated Groups, IT907-16) and by the University of Basque Country UPV/EHU (predoctoral grant PIF17/79). Authors wish to thank the intellectual and technical assistance from the ICTS "NANBIOSIS," more specifically by the Drug Formulation Unit (U10) of the CIBER in Bioengineering, Biomaterials, and Nanomedicine (CIBER-BBN) at the University of the Basque Country (UPV/EHU).

Author details

Myriam Sainz-Ramos[1,2†], Nuseibah AL Qtaish[1,2†], Idoia Gallego[1,2], Ilia Villate-Beitia[1,2], Tania López[1,2], Gustavo Puras[1,2*] and José Luis Pedraz[1,2*]

*Address all correspondence to: joseluis.pedraz@ehu.eus and gustavo.puras@ehu.eus

1 NanoBioCel Group, University of the Basque Country (UPV/EHU), Spain

2 Biomedical Research Networking Centre in Bioengineering, Biomaterials and Nanomedicine (CIBER-BBN), Vitoria-Gasteiz, Spain

† These authors contributed equally to the work.

References

[1] Wang Y, Wrennall JA, Cai Z, Li H, Mint SDN. Understanding how cystic fibrosis mutations disrupt CFTR function: From single molecules to animal models. The International Journal of Biochemistry & Cell Biology. 2014;**52**:47-57. DOI: 10.1016/j.biocel.2014.04.001

[2] Ronan NJ, Elborn JS, Plant BJ. Current and emerging comorbidities in cystic fibrosis. La Presse Médicale. 2017;**46**(6, Part 2):e138. DOI: 10.1016/j.lpm.2017.05.011

[3] Lane MA, Doe SJ. A new era in the treatment of cystic fibrosis. Clinical Medicine. 2014; **14**(1):76-78. DOI: 10.7861/clinmedicine.14-1-76

[4] Edwards J, Clarke A, Mint GD. Adults with cystic fibrosis—Responding to a new ageing population. Chronic Illness. 2013;**9**(4):312-319. DOI: 10.1177/1742395313479982

[5] Davies JC, Ebdon A, Mint OC. Recent advances in the management of cystic fibrosis. Archives of Disease in Childhood. 2014;**99**(11):1033-1036. DOI: 10.1136/archdischild-2013-304400

[6] Mayrhofer P, Schleef M, Mint JW. Use of minicircle plasmids for gene therapy. Gene Therapy of Cancer. 2009;**542**:87-104. DOI: 10.1007/978-1-59745-561-9_4

[7] McLachlan G, Davidson H, Holder E, Davies LA, Pringle IA, Sumner-Jones SG, et al. Preclinical evaluation of three non-viral gene transfer agents for cystic fibrosis after aerosol delivery to the ovine lung. Gene Therapy. 2011;**18**(10):996. DOI: 10.1038/gt.2011.55

[8] Griesenbach U, Alton E. Moving forward: Cystic fibrosis gene therapy. Human Molecular Genetics. 2013;**22**(R1):R58. DOI: 10.1093/hmg/ddt372

[9] Lodish H, Berk A, Zipursky SL, Matsudaira P, Baltimore D, Darnell J. DNA cloning with plasmid vectors. Molecular Cell Biology. 4th edition. New York: W. H. Freeman; 2000. Section 7.1

[10] Thibault T, Degrouard J, Baril P, Pichon C, Midoux P, Mint MJ. Production of DNA minicircles less than 250 base pairs through a novel concentrated DNA circularization assay enabling minicircle design with NF-κB inhibition activity. Nucleic Acids Research. 2017;**45**(5):e26. DOI: 10.1093/nar/gkw1034

[11] Yew NS, Zhao H, Wu I, Song A, Tousignant JD, Przybylska M, et al. Reduced inflammatory response to plasmid DNA vectors by elimination and inhibition of immunostimulatory CpG motifs. Molecular Therapy. 2000;**1**(3):255-262. DOI: 10.1006/mthe.2000.0036

[12] McLachlan G, Stevenson BJ, Davidson DJ, Porteous DJ. Bacterial DNA is implicated in the inflammatory response to delivery of DNA/DOTAP to mouse lungs. Gene Therapy. 2000;**7**(5):384. DOI: 10.1038/sj.gt.3301097

[13] Gill DR, Pringle IA, Mint HSC. Progress and prospects: The design and production of plasmid vectors. Gene Therapy. 2009;**16**(2):165. DOI: 10.1038/gt.2008.183

[14] Gaspar V, Melo-Diogo D, Costa E, Moreira A, Queiroz J, Pichon C, et al. Minicircle DNA vectors for gene therapy: Advances and applications. Expert Opinion on Biological Therapy. 2015;**15**(3):353-379. DOI: 10.1517/14712598.2015.996544

[15] Kay MA, He C, Mint CZ. A robust system for production of minicircle DNA vectors. Nature Biotechnology. 2010;**28**(12):1287. DOI: 10.1038/nbt.1708

[16] Ahmad-Nejad P, Häcker H, Rutz M, Bauer S, Vabulas R, Wagner H. Bacterial CpG-DNA and lipopolysaccharides activate Toll-like receptors at distinct cellular compartments. European Journal of Immunology. 2002;**32**(7):1958-1968. DOI: AID-IMMU1958> 3.0.CO;2-U

[17] Gracey Maniar LE, Maniar JM, Chen Z, Lu J, Fire AZ, Kay MA. Minicircle DNA vectors achieve sustained expression reflected by active chromatin and transcriptional level. Molecular Therapy. 2013;**21**(1):131-138. DOI: 10.1038/mt.2012.244

[18] Montier T, Delépine P, Pichon C, Férec C, Porteous DJ, Midoux P. Non-viral vectors in cystic fibrosis gene therapy: Progress and challenges. Trends in Biotechnology. 2004; **22**(11):586-592. DOI: 10.1016/j.tibtech.2004.09.009

[19] Alton EWFW, Armstrong DK, Ashby D, Bayfield KJ, Bilton D, Bloomfield EV, et al. Repeated nebulisation of non-viral CFTR gene therapy in patients with cystic fibrosis: A randomised, double-blind, placebo-controlled, phase 2b trial. The Lancet Respiratory Medicine. 2015;**3**(9):684-691. DOI: 10.1016/S2213-2600(15)00245-3

[20] Villate-Beitia I, Zarate J, Puras G, Pedraz JL. Gene delivery to the lungs: Pulmonary gene therapy for cystic fibrosis. Drug Development and Industrial Pharmacy. 2017;**43**(7):1071-1081. DOI: 10.1080/03639045.2017.1298122

[21] Kim YG, Cha J, Chandrasegaran S. Hybrid restriction enzymes: Zinc finger fusions to Fok I cleavage domain. Proceedings of the National Academy of Sciences of the United States of America. 1996;**93**(3):1156-1160

[22] Lee CM, Flynn R, Hollywood JA, Scallan MF, Harrison PT. Correction of the ΔF508 mutation in the cystic fibrosis transmembrane conductance regulator gene by zinc-finger nuclease homology-directed repair. Biores Open Access. 2012;**1**(3):99-108. DOI: 10.1089/biores.2012.0218

[23] Crane A, Kramer P, Bui J, Chung W, Li X, Gonzalez-Garay M, et al. Targeted correction and restored function of the CFTR gene in cystic fibrosis induced pluripotent stem cells. Stem Cell Reports. 2015;**4**(4):569-577. DOI: 10.1016/j.stemcr.2015.02.005

[24] Kormann MSD. In vivo gene correction of cystic fibrosis. In: Cystic Fibrosis in the Light of New Research. InTech; 2015. DOI: 10.5772/60697

[25] Reyon D, Tsai SQ, Khayter C, Foden JA, Sander JD, Joung JK. FLASH assembly of TALENs for high-throughput genome editing. Nature Biotechnology. 2012;**30**(5):460. DOI: 10. 1038/nbt.2170

[26] Camarasa MV, Gálvez VM. Robust method for TALEN-edited correction of pF508del in patient-specific induced pluripotent stem cells. Stem Cell Research & Therapy. 2016;**7**: 1-27. DOI: 10.1186/s13287-016-0275-6

[27] Mojica FJM, Montoliu L. On the origin of CRISPR-Cas technology: From prokaryotes to mammals. Trends in Microbiology. 2016;**24**(10):811-820. DOI: 10.1016/j.tim.2016.06.005

[28] Dominguez AA, Lim WA, Qi LS. Beyond editing: Repurposing CRISPR–Cas9 for precision genome regulation and interrogation. Nature Reviews. Molecular Cell Biology. 2016;**17**(1):5-15. DOI: 10.1038/nrm.2015.2

[29] Schwank G, Koo B, Sasselli V, Dekkers J, Heo I, Demircan T, et al. Functional repair of CFTR by CRISPR/Cas9 in intestinal stem cell organoids of cystic fibrosis patients. Cell Stem Cell. 2013;**13**(6):653-658. DOI: 10.1016/j.stem.2013.11.002

[30] Rolland A. Gene medicines: The end of the beginning? Advanced Drug Delivery Reviews. 2005;**57**(5):669-673. DOI: 10.1016/j.addr.2005.01.002

[31] Aliño SF, Bobadilla M, Crespo J, Lejarreta M. Human α1-antitrypsin gene transfer to in vivo mouse hepatocytes. Human Gene Therapy. 1996;**7**(4):531-536. DOI: 10.1089/hum.1996.7.4-531

[32] Zabner J, Couture LA, Gregory RJ, Graham SM, Smith AE, Welsh MJ. Adenovirus-mediated gene transfer transiently corrects the chloride transport defect in nasal epithelia of patients with cystic fibrosis. Cell. 1993;**75**(2):207-216. DOI: 10.1016/0092-8674(93)80063-K

[33] Duan D, Sharma P, Yang J, Yue Y, Dudus L, Zhang Y, et al. Circular intermediates of recombinant adeno-associated virus have defined structural characteristics responsible for long-term episomal persistence in muscle tissue. Journal of Virology. 1998; **72**(11):8568-8577

[34] Schnepp BC, Jensen RL, Chen C, Johnson PR, Clark KR. Characterization of adeno-associated virus genomes isolated from human tissues. Journal of Virology. 2005;**79**(23):14793-14803. DOI: 10.1128/JVI.79.23.14793-14803.2005

[35] Chamberlain K, Riyad JM, Weber T. Expressing transgenes that exceed the packaging capacity of adeno-associated virus capsids. Human Gene Therapy Methods. 2016;**27**(1):1-12. DOI: 10.1089/hgtb.2015.140

[36] Moss RB, Rodman D, Spencer LT, Aitken ML, Zeitlin PL, Waltz D, et al. Repeated adeno-associated virus serotype 2 aerosol-mediated cystic fibrosis transmembrane regulator gene transfer to the lungs of patients with cystic fibrosis: A multicenter, double-blind, placebo-controlled trial. Chest. 2004;**125**(2):509-521. DOI: 10.1378/chest.125.2.509

[37] Moss RB, Milla C, Colombo J, Accurso F, Zeitlin PL, Clancy JP, et al. Repeated aerosolized AAV-CFTR for treatment of cystic fibrosis: A randomized placebo-controlled phase 2B trial. Human Gene Therapy. 2007;**18**(8):726-732. DOI: 10.1089/hum.2007.022

[38] Faust SM, Bell P, Cutler BJ, Ashley SN, Zhu Y, Rabinowitz JE, et al. CpG-depleted adeno-associated virus vectors evade immune detection. Journal of Clinical Investigation. 2013;**123**(7):2994. DOI: 10.1172/JCI68205

[39] Mays LE, Wang L, Tenney R, Bell P, Nam H, Lin J, et al. Mapping the structural determinants responsible for enhanced T cell activation to the immunogenic adeno-associated virus capsid from isolate rhesus 32.33. Journal of Virology. 2013;**87**(17):9473-9485. DOI: 10.1128/JVI.00596-13

[40] Stocker AG, Kremer KL, Koldej R, Miller DS, Anson DS, Parsons DW. Single-dose lentiviral gene transfer for lifetime airway gene expression. The Journal of Gene Medicine. 2009;**11**(10):861-867. DOI: 10.1002/jgm.1368

[41] Griesenbach U, Inoue M, Meng C, Farley R, Chan M, Newman NK, et al. Assessment of F/HN-pseudotyped lentivirus as a clinically relevant vector for lung gene therapy. American Journal of Respiratory and Critical Care Medicine. 2012;**186**(9):846-856. DOI: 10.1164/rccm.201206-1056OC

[42] Cooney AL, Abou Alaiwa MH, Shah VS, Bouzek DC, Stroik MR, Powers LS, et al. Lentiviral-mediated phenotypic correction of cystic fibrosis pigs. JCI Insight. 2016;**1**(14):1-9. DOI: 10.1172/jci.insight.88730

[43] Alton EWFW, Beekman JM, Boyd AC, Brand J, Carlon MS, Connolly MM, et al. Preparation for a first-in-man lentivirus trial in patients with cystic fibrosis. Thorax. 2017; **72**(2):137-147. DOI: 10.1136/thoraxjnl-2016-208406

[44] Yin H, Kanasty RL, Eltoukhy AA, Vegas AJ, Dorkin JR, Anderson DG. Non-viral vectors for gene-based therapy. Nature Reviews Genetics. 2014;**15**(8):541. DOI: 10.1038/nrg3763

[45] Davis ME. Non-viral gene delivery systems. Current Opinion in Biotechnology. 2002; **13**(2):128-131. DOI: 10.1016/S0958-1669(02)00294-X

[46] Keles E, Song Y, Du D, Dong W, Lin Y. Recent progress in nanomaterials for gene delivery applications. Biomaterials Science. 2016;**4**(9):1291-1309. DOI: 10.1039/C6BM00441E

[47] Kinsey BM, Orson CLD, Orson FM. Non-viral gene delivery to the lungs. Current Gene Therapy. 2005;**5**(2):181-194. DOI: 10.2174/1566523053544254

[48] Al-Dosari MS, Gao X. Nonviral gene delivery: Principle, limitations, and recent progress. The AAPS Journal. 2009;**11**(4):1-35. DOI: 10.1208/s12248-009-9143-y

[49] Pringle IA, Hyde SC, Gill DR. Non-viral vectors in cystic fibrosis gene therapy: Recent developments and future prospects. Expert Opinion on Biological Therapy. 2009;**9**(8):991-1003. DOI: 10.1517/14712590903055029

[50] Grosse S, Aron Y, Honoré I, Thévenot G, Danel C, Roche A, et al. Lactosylated polyethylenimine for gene transfer into airway epithelial cells: Role of the sugar moiety in cell delivery and intracellular trafficking of the complexes. The Journal of Gene Medicine. 2004;**6**(3):345-356. DOI: 10.1002/jgm.515

[51] Eastman SJ, Lukason MJ, Tousignant JD, Murray H, Lane MD, George JAS, et al. Mint: A concentrated and stable aerosol formulation of cationic lipid: DNA complexes giving high-level gene expression in mouse lung. Human Gene Therapy. 1997;**8**(6):765-773. DOI: 10.1089/hum.1997.8.6-765

[52] Alton E, Stern M, Farley R, Jaffe A, Chadwick SL, Phillips J, et al. Cationic lipid-mediated CFTR gene transfer to the lungs and nose of patients with cystic fibrosis: A double-blind placebo-controlled trial. The Lancet. 1999;**353**(9157):947-954. DOI: 10.1016/S0140-6736(98)06532-5

[53] Villate-Beitia I, Puras G, Zarate J, Agirre M, Ojeda E, Pedraz JL. First insights into non-invasive administration routes for non-viral gene therapy. In: Gene Therapy—Principles and Challenges. InTech; 2015. DOI: 10.5772/61060

[54] Agirre M, Zarate J, Puras G, Rojas LA, Alemany R, Pedraz JL. Strategies for improving the systemic delivery of oncolytic adenoviruses and plasmids: Potential application of non-viral carriers. In: Atta-ur-Rahman M, Chouldhary I, editors. Frontiers in Anti-Cancer Drug Discovery. Bentham Science; 2013. pp. 190-225

[55] Parhiz H, Hashemi M, Ramezani M. Non-biological gene carriers designed for overcoming the major extra- and intracellular hurdles in gene delivery, an updated review. Nanomedicine Journal. 2015;**2**(1):1-20. DOI: 10.7508/nmj.2015.01.001

[56] Amoozgar Z, Yeo Y. Recent advances in stealth coating of nanoparticle drug delivery systems. Wiley Interdisciplinary Reviews. Nanomedicine and Nanobiotechnology. 2012;**4**(2):219-233. DOI: 10.1002/wnan.1157

[57] Ishihara T, Maeda T, Sakamoto H, Takasaki N, Shigyo M, Ishida T, et al. Evasion of the accelerated blood clearance phenomenon by coating of nanoparticles with various hydrophilic polymers. Biomacromolecules. 2010;**11**(10):2700-2706. DOI: 10.1021/bm100754e

[58] Sanders N, Rudolph C, Braeckmans K, De Smedt SC, Demeester J. Extracellular barriers in respiratory gene therapy. Advanced Drug Delivery Reviews. 2009;**61**(2):115-127. DOI: 10.1016/j.addr.2008.09.011

[59] King M, Rubin BK. Pharmacological approaches to discovery and development of new mucolytic agents. Advanced Drug Delivery Reviews. 2002;**54**(11):1475-1490. DOI: 10.1016/S0169-409X(02)00156-4

[60] Medina-Kauwe LK, Xie J, Hamm-Alvarez S. Intracellular trafficking of nonviral vectors. Gene Therapy. 2005;**12**(24):1734. DOI: 10.1038/sj.gt.3302592

[61] Xiang S, Tong H, Shi Q, Fernandes JC, Jin T, Dai K, et al. Uptake mechanisms of non-viral gene delivery. Journal of Controlled Release. 2012;**158**(3):371-378. DOI: 10.1016/j.jconrel.2011.09.093

[62] Hillaireau H, Couvreur P. Nanocarriers' entry into the cell: Relevance to drug delivery. Cellular and Molecular Life Sciences. 2009;**66**(17):2873-2896. DOI: 10.1007/s00018-009-0053-z

[63] Khalil IA, Kogure K, Akita H, Harashima H. Uptake pathways and subsequent intracellular trafficking in nonviral gene delivery. Pharmacological Reviews. 2006;**58**(1):32-45. DOI: 10.1124/pr.58.1.8

[64] Varkouhi AK, Scholte M, Storm G, Haisma HJ. Endosomal escape pathways for delivery of biologicals. Journal of Controlled Release. 2011;**151**(3):220-228. DOI: 10.1016/j.jconrel.2010.11.004

[65] Kiss AL, Botos E. Endocytosis via caveolae: Alternative pathway with distinct cellular compartments to avoid lysosomal degradation? Journal of Cellular and Molecular Medicine. 2009;**13**(7):1228-1237. DOI: 10.1111/j.1582-4934.2009.00754.x

[66] Delgado D, del Pozo-Rodríguez A, Solinís MÁ, Rodríguez-Gascón A. Understanding the mechanism of protamine in solid lipid nanoparticle-based lipofection: The importance of the entry pathway. European Journal of Pharmaceutics and Biopharmaceutics. 2011;**79**(3):495-502. DOI: 10.1016/j.ejpb.2011.06.005

[67] Jans DA, Hubner S. Regulation of protein transport to the nucleus: Central role of phosphorylation. Physiological Reviews. 1996;**76**(3):651-685. DOI: 10.1152/physrev.1996.76.3.651

[68] de Kruijf W, Ehrhardt C. Inhalation delivery of complex drugs—The next steps. Current Opinion in Pharmacology. 2017;**36**:52-57. DOI: 10.1016/j.coph.2017.07.015

[69] Lentz YK, Worden LR, Anchordoquy TJ, Lengsfeld CS. Effect of jet nebulization on DNA: Identifying the dominant degradation mechanism and mitigation methods. Journal of Aerosol Science. 2005;**36**(8):973-990. DOI: 10.1016/j.jaerosci.2004.11.017

[70] Jr DJC, Fogg JM, Ii DES, Gilbert BE, Zechiedrich L. Supercoiled minivector DNA resists shear forces associated with gene therapy delivery. Gene Therapy. 2012;**19**(1):94. DOI: 10.1038/gt.2011.77

[71] Gharse S, Fiegel J. Large porous hollow particles: Lightweight champions of pulmonary drug delivery. Current Pharmaceutical Design. 2016;**22**(17):2463-2469

[72] Patton JS, Brain JD, Davies LA, Fiegel J, Gumbleton M, Kim K, et al. The particle has landed—Characterizing the fate of inhaled pharmaceuticals. Journal of Aerosol Medicine and Pulmonary Drug Delivery. 2010;**23**(S2):71. DOI: 10.1089/jamp.2010.0836

[73] Griesenbach U, McLachlan G, Owaki T, Somerton L, Shu T, Baker A, et al. Validation of recombinant Sendai virus in a non-natural host model. Gene Therapy. 2011;**18**(2):182. DOI: 10.1038/gt.2010.131

[74] Hida K, Lai SK, Suk JS, Won SY, Boyle MP, Hanes J. Common gene therapy viral vectors do not efficiently penetrate sputum from cystic fibrosis patients. PLoS One. 2011; **6**(5):e19919. DOI: 10.1371/journal.pone.0019919

[75] Laube BL. Aerosolized medications for gene and peptide therapy. Respiratory Care. 2015;**60**(6):806-824. DOI: 10.4187/respcare.03554

[76] LGd R, Svolos M, Hartwig B, Windhab N, Young PM, Traini D. Inhaled gene delivery: A formulation and delivery approach. Expert Opinion on Drug Delivery. 2017;**14**(3): 319-330. DOI: 10.1080/17425247.2016.1214569

[77] Ari A. Jet, ultrasonic, and mesh nebulizers: An evaluation of nebulizers for better clinical outcomes. Eurasian Journal of Pulmonology. 2014;**16**(1):1-7. DOI: 10.5152/ejp.2014.00087

[78] Dailey LA, Kleemann E, Merdan T, Petersen H, Schmehl T, Gessler T, et al. Modified polyethylenimines as non viral gene delivery systems for aerosol therapy: Effects of nebulization on cellular uptake and transfection efficiency. Journal of Controlled Release. 2004; **100**(3):425-436. DOI: 10.1016/j.jconrel.2004.08.031

[79] Mohammed-Saeid W, Michel D, El-Aneed A, Verrall RE, Low NH, Badea I. Development of lyophilized Gemini surfactant-based gene delivery systems: Influence of lyophilization on the structure, activity and stability of the lipoplexes. Journal of Pharmacy & Pharmaceutical Sciences. 2012;**15**(4):548-567

[80] Seville PC, Kellaway IW, Birchall JC. Preparation of dry powder dispersions for non-viral gene delivery by freeze-drying and spray-drying. The Journal of Gene Medicine. 2002;**4**(4):428-437. DOI: 10.1002/jgm.282

[81] Liang W, Kwok PCL, Chow MYT, Tang P, Mason AJ, Chan H, et al. Formulation of pH responsive peptides as inhalable dry powders for pulmonary delivery of nucleic acids. European Journal of Pharmaceutics and Biopharmaceutics. 2014;**86**(1):64-73. DOI: 10. 1016/j.ejpb.2013.05.006

[82] Kuo JS. The effect of protective agents on the stability of plasmid DNA by the process of spray-drying. Journal of Pharmacy and Pharmacology. 2003;**55**(3):301-306. DOI: 10. 1211/002235702702

[83] Pfeifer C, Hasenpusch G, Uezguen S, Aneja MK, Reinhardt D, Kirch J, et al. Dry powder aerosols of polyethylenimine (PEI)-based gene vectors mediate efficient gene delivery to the lung. Journal of Controlled Release. 2011;**154**(1):69-76. DOI: 10.1016/j. jconrel.2011.05.006

[84] Mohajel N, Najafabadi AR, Azadmanesh K, Amini M, Vatanara A, Moazeni E, et al. Mint: Drying of a plasmid containing formulation: Chitosan as a protecting agent. Daru. 2012; **20**(1):22. DOI: 10.1186/2008-2231-20-22

[85] Tsukamoto M, Okuda T, Okamoto H, Higuchi Y, Kawakami S, Yamashita F, et al. Bovine serum albumin as a lyoprotectant for preparation of DNA dry powder formulations using the spray-freeze drying method. Biological & Pharmaceutical Bulletin. 2012; **35**(7):1178-1181

[86] Flory E, Reinhardt J. European regulatory tools for advanced therapy medicinal products. Transfusion Medicine and Hemotherapy. 2013;**40**(6):409-412. DOI: 10.1159/000356364

[87] (cat) The Committee for Advanced TherapiesSchneider CK, Salmikangas P, Jilma B, Flamion B, Todorova LR, et al. Mint: Challenges with advanced therapy medicinal products and how to meet them. Nature Reviews Drug Discovery. 2010;**9**(3):195. DOI: 10.1038/nrd3052

[88] Jaffé A, Prasad SA, Larcher V, Hart S. Gene therapy for children with cystic fibrosis—Who has the right to choose? Journal of Medical Ethics. 2006;**32**(6):361-364. DOI: 10.1136/ jme.2005.012740

[89] Davies LA, Nunez-Alonso GA, Hebel HL, Scheule RK, Cheng SH, Hyde SC, et al. A novel mixing device for the reproducible generation of nonviral gene therapy formulations. BioTechniques. 2010;**49**(3):666-668. DOI: 10.2144/000113498

Chapter 3

Mechanisms for Controlling HIV-1 Infection: A Gene Therapy Approach

Katherine Ognenovska, Vera Klemm, Scott Ledger,
Stuart Turville, Geoff Symonds,
Anthony D. Kelleher and Chantelle L. Ahlenstiel

Additional information is available at the end of the chapter

http://dx.doi.org/10.5772/intechopen.79669

Abstract

Current anti-retroviral treatment (ART) for HIV-1 is highly effectively at controlling the infection. However, during early infection the virus establishes a latent reservoir, which is not impacted by ART. Any treatment interruption rapidly results in virus rebound from the latent reservoir to pre-therapy levels and thus ART does not constitute an HIV-1 cure. Alternate treatments are currently being explored in the form of gene therapy, following the success of the Berlin patient who has had undetectable virus since 2007. This review will describe the contrasting cure approaches that are currently the focus of multiple studies to control HIV, then focus in on functional cure gene therapy strategies; specifically, epigenetic silencing of HIV-1 by various methods, including RNA-directed transcriptional gene silencing. The various delivery strategies for targeting cells of the latent reservoir will be reviewed and finally, the clinical status and current challenges for *ex vivo* versus *in vivo* gene therapy delivery approaches will be discussed.

Keywords: HIV, functional cure, "block and lock", epigenetic silencing, si/shRNA, latent reservoir, gene therapy

1. Introduction

HIV-1 was first identified in the 1980s and currently infects ~37 million people world-wide [1]. There has been a concerted global effort in strategic planning for HIV prevention, with the current goals in multiple countries for the end of 2020 being to significantly reduce or virtually eliminate new infections. This goal is based on the increased uptake and availability of anti-retroviral therapy (ART) and the more recent pre-exposure prophylaxis (PrEP), which has been embraced by many countries, particularly the US, UK and Australia [2], and demonstrated in landmark studies to prevent transmission by 99% [3, 4]. Additionally, the recent OPPOSITES ATTRACT study [5, 6] and PARTNER study [7] both showed that ART effectively reduces that rate of transmission to zero in homosexual male serodiscordant couples.

However, while ART is highly effectively at controlling HIV-1 infection, it does not impact the latent reservoir, which is established early during virus infection. This allows the latent virus to recrudesce following any treatment interruption and results in rapid virus rebound to pre-therapy levels. Therefore, ART does not constitute an HIV-1 cure. As is the case for many other diseases, gene therapy is being explored as an alternate HIV-1 treatment. There are, however, challenges specific to HIV, that may not arise in gene therapy approaches for other diseases. In the context of HIV, the latent reservoir represents a major barrier for developing an HIV cure, since ART has no effect on the integrated provirus and there is currently lack of a biomarker to identify cells that carry latent virus. Combined with the inability to identify latent cells and the rare frequency of latently-infected cells (~1 in 10^6 cells) these hurdles make the development of a gene delivery platform uniquely challenging, especially in terms of a systemic *in vivo* approach. Another difficulty is that not all integrated provirus is the same, with some being full-length intact genomes and others being defective genomes that carry large deletions and will not result in productive infection following reactivation [8]. These are the barriers that must be addressed to ensure a gene therapy approach to HIV translates into patient outcomes. The unique challenges facing HIV-1 gene therapy and current solutions are described in this chapter.

2. HIV-1 life cycle: challenges for an HIV-1 cure

HIV-1 can infect a wide range of cells, predominantly targeting $CD4^+$ T cells, dendritic cells, macrophages and other myeloid lineage cells [9]. This is achieved by binding of the viral envelope glycoprotein gp120 to the CD4 receptor, triggering a conformational change that allows for CCR5 or CXCR4 coreceptor binding. Further conformational changes in gp41 initiate a membrane fusion reaction that allows the viral capsid cytoplasmic entry [10]. Upon entry, the capsid disassembles to release viral RNA and proteins. To protect this genetic material, host restriction factors are subverted. With the aid of commandeered host cell machinery, a reverse transcription complex is formed and complementary viral DNA (cDNA) generated. The resulting pre-integration complex is transported via cytoskeletal manipulation to a nuclear pore complex where it is actively imported. The ability to traverse the nuclear membrane allows HIV to productively infect non-dividing cells. Viral integrase then facilitates the integration of viral DNA into the host genome to form the provirus [11]. Thus, HIV tethers its survival to the longevity of the cell and establishes the latent provirus reservoir, from which virus can reactivate. Using host replication machinery, viral RNA is then transcribed and exported to the cytoplasm. Proteins required for infectivity are synthesised and trafficked to the plasma membrane. Along with two RNA copies of the HIV genome, these proteins are assembled and packaged into immature virions in a process mediated by the viral Gag polyprotein. Once released from the plasma membrane, viral protease cleaves Gag into three structural proteins to create the mature infectious virion [12]. The HIV-1 life cycle is summarised in **Figure 1**.

http://dx.doi.org/10.5772/intechopen.79669

While the above cycle is the most common model of HIV-1 infection, it is not exclusive. Numerous alternate pathways at varying stages of infection have been observed. For example, rather than the release of free HIV-1 virions, cell-to-cell transmission via infectious synapses can occur [13]. This modification is a more efficient means of infectivity [14]. Additionally, the above model does not account for infection of the central nervous system [15], in particular cells such as astrocytes, which lack the CD4 receptor [16]. While some of the proposed pathways remain controversial, HIV-1 is undeniably a versatile virus capable of hijacking diverse systems. The infectious route it takes may depend on the cell type, its available resources and activation status.

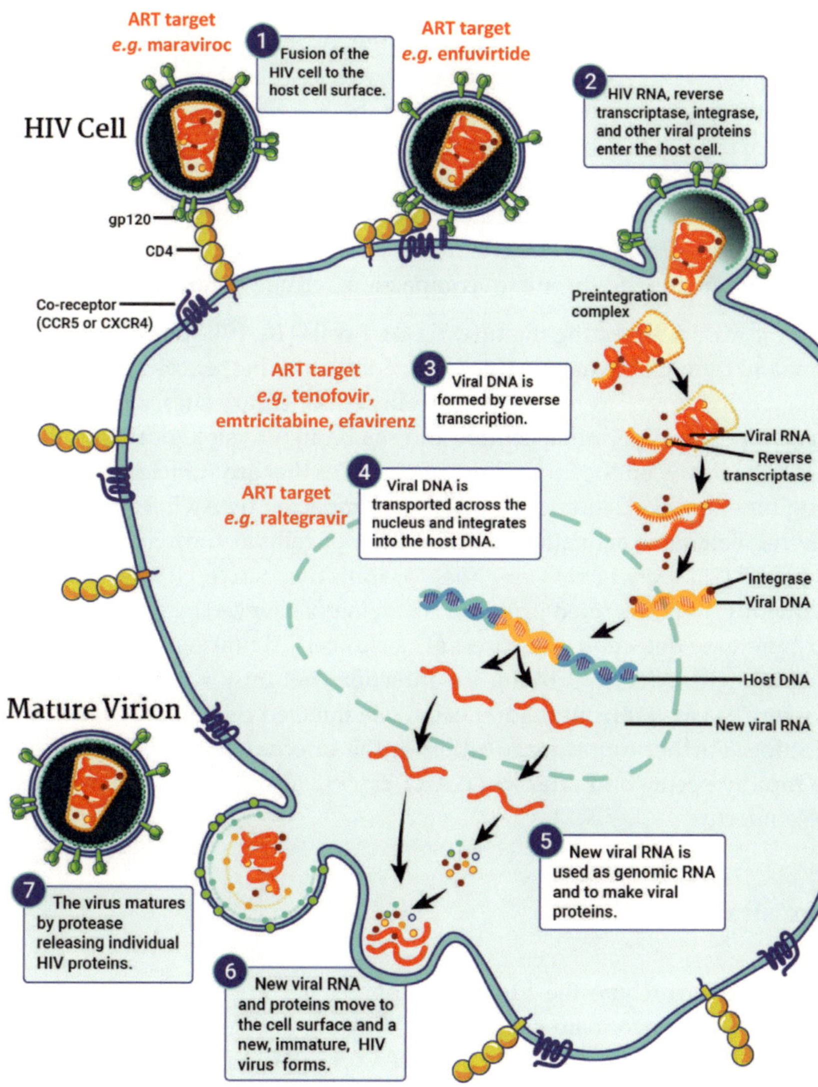

Figure 1. HIV-1 life cycle and stages targeted by antiretroviral therapy (ART). ART drugs target various stages of the HIV life cycle, with some common drugs shown. Credit: National Institute of Allergy and Infectious Diseases (NIAID).

2.1. The Life cycle and ART treatment

Due to the inherent sequence variability of HIV-1 and the ability for virus resistance to arise, multiple stages in the virus life cycle need to be targeted by ART to control the infection. As illustrated in **Figure 1**, stages that are targeted can include binding, fusion, reverse transcriptions and integration, among others, with either one or more ART drugs from each stage being utilised to provide sufficient HIV-1 control. An example of one such drug combination is TRUVADA®, which combines two drugs targeting the reverse transcription stage, emtricitabine and tenofovir and has been widely embraced for PrEP treatment.

2.2. The latent reservoir

Although the versatility of HIV-1 presents a challenge for the development of therapeutics, by far, the latent cellular reservoirs are the greatest barrier to developing a cure. The difficulties in controlling these virus reservoirs arise when the infection becomes latent. While the exact mechanisms of HIV latency are still being precisely defined, studies have demonstrated epigenetic regulation is involved in suppressing virus transcription, with the presence of classic epigenetic repressive marks, including methylation (*i.e.* histone 3 lysine 27 trimethylation (H3K27me3)) and deacetylation (*i.e.* Histone deacetylase 1 (HDAC1)) on N-terminal histone tails inducing specific epigenetic chromatin compaction, termed heterochromatin [17].

The latent reservoir resides in resting memory CD4+ T cells [18, 19], such as central memory, effector memory and transitional memory cells [8], T follicular helper cells [20], macrophages and other myeloid cells, as well as in immune privileged sanctuary sites, such as the gut [21], lymph nodes and associated germinal centers and the brain. Physiologically, in their resting states CD4+ T cells have low endocytic and metabolic rates that are sufficient for maintenance of housekeeping functions [22]. As such, they are not impacted by ART. To retain dormancy, they negatively regulate gene activation via inhibition of cellular transcription factors, such as NF-κB and NFAT [23]: host factors essential for initiating active HIV-1 virus production [24–26]. Consequently, the integrated provirus is reversibly silenced by epigenetic repression and evades host immune detection. This presents a clinically daunting prospect. As memory cells are long lived, with ART controlling the infection, not only would eradication of the reservoir take over 70 years [18], but theoretically, one infected cell could sufficiently sustain a life-long infection. Further, upon reactivation of the infected cell/s by any stimuli, virus recrudescence rapidly occurs and thus while ART can effectively control HIV-1 infection, it does not represent a cure.

3. HIV-1 cure strategies

Various approaches to overcome the viral reservoir barrier are being pursued. Primarily, they can be separated into two main categories: sterilising and functional. Both approaches aim for an undetectable viral load without the need for ART, with the sterilising approach being defined as complete eradication of the virus, and conversely, the functional approach is defined as controlling the virus reservoir without its eradication.

3.1. Shock and kill

The most studied sterilising approach is aptly named "shock and kill". This concept explores the use of *latency reversing agents* (LRAs) to "shock" the virus into reactivation, whereby it is detected and "killed" by either its own cytotoxicity or the host immune system. To date, this purging strategy has been largely unsuccessful. Proposed agents either induce global immune reactivation, leading to increased pro-inflammatory cytokines and severe side effects, or *in vitro* efficacy has simply failed to translate *in vivo* [27–32]. Extensive descriptions of LRAs and the next step of optimising the "kill" step is reviewed by Kim et al., [33] and are not the focus of this chapter. However, one recent study has demonstrated a specific kill response mediated by ricin A, which is initially encapsulated in a novel nanocapsule polymer shell and then activated and released via the ricin A peptide crosslinkers being cleaved by HIV-1 protease [34]. Some of the LRAs under investigation are summarised in **Table 1** and a schematic of the process is shown in **Figure 2**.

3.2. Block and lock

The limited success of sterilising cures has shifted the priority to identifying a functional cure; which is now seen as a more realistic approach to controlling the viral reservoir, without ART. The functional cure approach is termed "block and lock". This concept exploits the use of *latency inducing agents* (LIAs) to "block" virus gene transcription at the promoter via epigenetic mechanisms and "lock" the integrated virus genome in a permanent super-latent state, which resembles the natural latent reservoir. We and others are pursuing this approach to provide a sustained virus remission, without ART. Some of the LIAs under investigation are summarised in **Table 1** and a schematic of the process is shown in **Figure 2**.

3.2.1. Tat-inhibitor didehydro-cortistatin A (dCA)

In 2012, the Valente group reported a novel small molecule inhibitor of HIV transcription, termed Didehydro-cortistatin A (dCA) [35]. Derived from a marine sponge, dCA inhibits Tat-mediated transactivation of integrated HIV provirus via disrupting binding of the transactivation response (TAR) element to Tat through direct binding competition with the RNA hairpin TAR-binding domain of Tat. Effectively disrupting the Tat/TAR complex, dCA induced prolonged suppression of virus transcription in HeLa-CD4 cells infected with HIV-$1_{NL4.3}$ for 2 months with constant treatment and out to a further 27 days following cessation of treatment, as determined by measuring viral RNA levels. The inhibitory effect of dCA on HIV replication *ex vivo* in primary CD4+ T cells isolated from eight HIV-1 infected individuals on suppressive ART was ~60% compared to no treatment, while ART treatment alone reduced viral production to ~40% and dCA treatment alone reduced virus production to ~25% [35]. The study reported there were no apparent cytotoxic effects in cell culture models or when assessed in C57Bl-6 mice at the concentrations used. Further optimisation of dCA will be required if the treatment is to be effective in the absence of ART, as desired for a functional HIV cure, and to increase the longevity of the suppressive effect.

Latency reversing agents (LRAs)	
Class	**Agent**
Epigenetic Modifiers	Histone deacetylase inhibitors (HDACs)
	Methylation inhibitors
	Methyl-transferase inhibitors
	Bromodomain inhibitors
	P-TEFb activators
Protein Kinase C Agonists	Prostratin/Bryostatin
	Ingenol B/PEP0005
PI3K/Akt pathway	Disulfiram
	STATS signalling benzotriazole
	mTOR complex Rapamycin
TCR Activators	Immune checkpoint blockers
Cytokines	IL-15
TLR Agonists	TLR7
	TLR9
Latency inducing agents (LIAs)	
Class	**Agent**
Epigenetic Modifiers	Didehydro-cortistatin A (dCA)
	siRNA
	shRNA
	Ubiquitin-like, containing PHD and RING finger domains 1 protein (UHRF1)
	Nullbasic
HIV Integrase inhibitors	LEDGINs

P-TEFb, positive transcription elongation factor b; TLR, Toll-like receptor; mTOR, mechanistic target of rapamycin; STAT5, signal transducer and activator of transcription 5; IL-15, interleukin-15; dCA, Didehydro-cortistatin A; UHRF1, Ubiquitin-like, containing PHD and RING finger domains 1 protein.

Table 1. Agents that modulate HIV latency.

3.2.2. RNA silencing

RNA interference (RNAi) is a fundamentally conserved process crucial for viral defence and the regulation of normal gene expression. Since its initial discovery in transgenic tobacco plants [36], the RNAi field has erupted with literature exploring the depth of its possibilities. From a tool to study basic gene functions, to a remedy for previously untreatable conditions, RNAi has the potential to revolutionise research and medicine. As a result, it has been extensively studied and characterised in a wide array of organisms, particularly plants (*Arabidopsis thaliana* [37, 38]), the nematode *Caenorhabditis elegans* [39] and fission yeast *Schizosaccharomyces pombe* (*S. pombe*) [40]. Two distinct pathways have since emerged: post-transcriptional gene silencing (PTGS) and transcriptional gene silencing (TGS); also termed epigenetic silencing (refer to **Figure 3** for an overview).

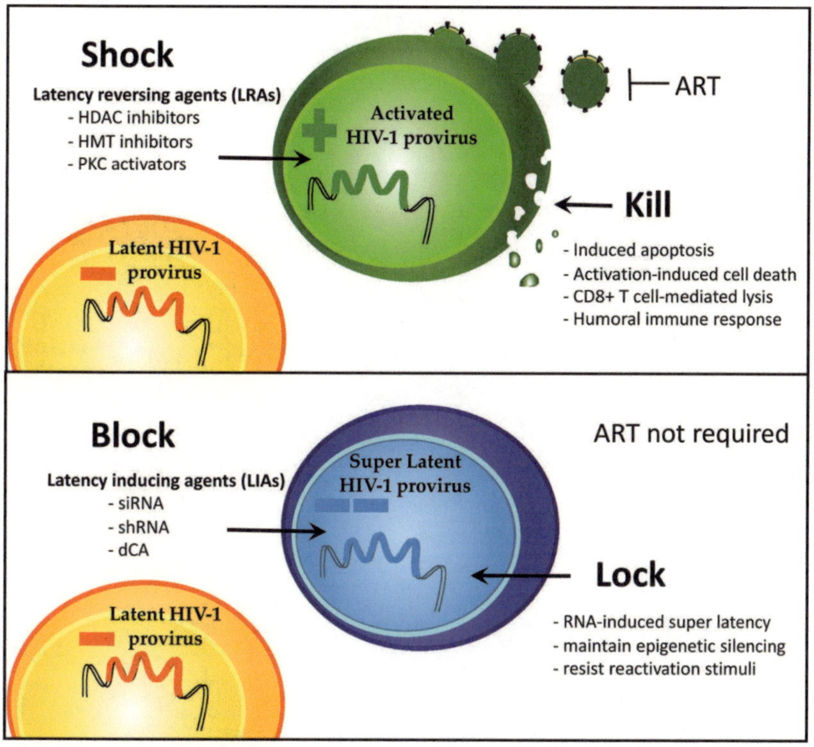

Figure 2. "Shock and kill" versus "Block and Lock" HIV cure strategies. Latency reversing agents (LRAs) activate or "shock" the HIV-1 provirus awake with the aim that the infected cell will then undergo "kill" via cytotoxic or host immune mechanisms. Latency inducing agents (LIAs) mediate the opposite effect, by "blocking" virus replication and "locking" the virus genome in an induced "super-latency" that is refractory to reactivation. HDAC, histone deacetylase; HMT, histone methyl transferase; PKC, protein kinase C; dCA, didehydro-cortistatin A; ART, antiretroviral therapy.

PTGS was the first distinct pathway to be discovered in 1998 by Fire and Mello [39]. It can be considered the predominantly cytoplasmic arm of RNAi. Briefly, short interfering RNAs (siRNAs) 19–23 base pairs long are processed by the Dicer endonuclease and loaded onto the Argonaute 2 (Ago2) protein. Several of other proteins are recruited to form the RNA-induced silencing complex (RISC). This complex uses the siRNA as complementary anti-sense guides to identify target mRNA in the cytoplasm that are subsequently cleaved and degraded by the catalytic activity of Ago2 [41]. As a result, target gene expression is transiently downregulated prior to translation. Exhibiting enormous potential, PTGS has since been developed as a tool to selectively inhibit the expression of critical HIV-1 viral proteins *in vitro,* leading to significant reductions in viral replication [42–46]. The sequence specific nature of the PTGS process suggests there are minimal off-target effects [47], although these can still occur. Some reports have shown that introducing exogenous siRNA less than 24 base pairs in length does not trigger an interferon mediated immune response or defence mechanism to the synthetic material [48].

While these are all highly desirable traits for future gene therapeutics, PTGS has several limitations, particularly in the context of HIV-1, which leave it unsuitable for gene therapy. A consequence of its high specificity is that a nucleotide mismatches between the siRNA and its target could be sufficient to abrogate silencing [49]. Hence, in the context of a highly diverse virus with multiple subtypes, a conserved target sequence must be carefully selected. Due

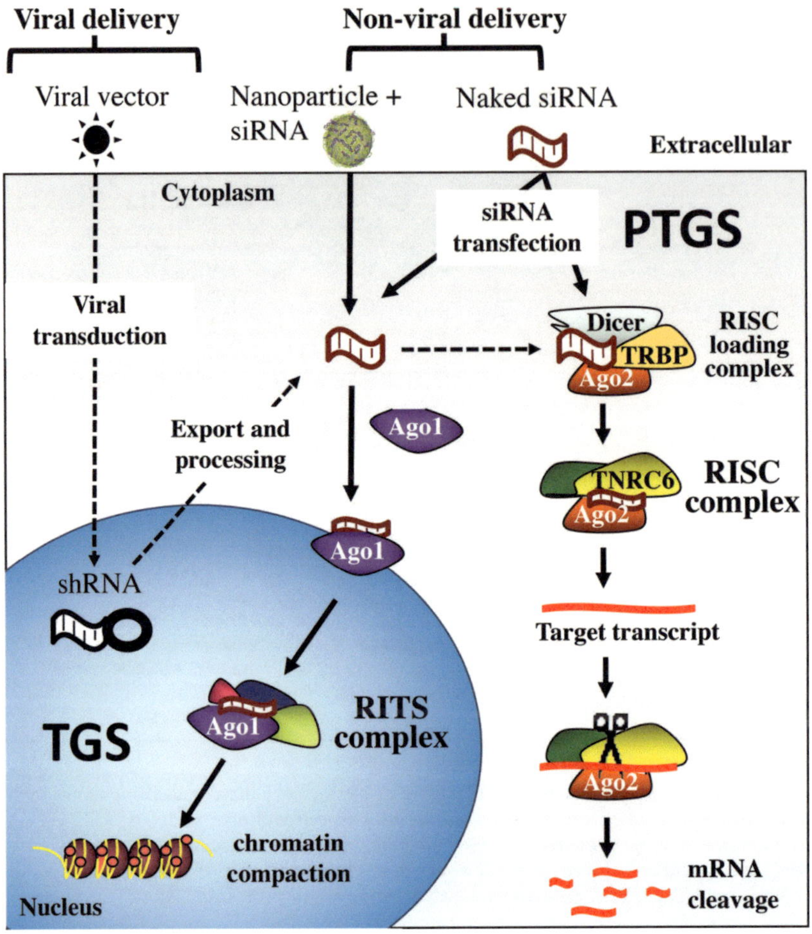

Figure 3. Gene silencing pathways mediated by siRNA. siRNA duplexes induce posttranscriptional gene silencing (PTGS) predominately in the cytoplasm through RISC machinery initiating mRNA degradation, and transcriptional gene silencing (TGS) in the nucleus through the RITS complex inducing chromatin compaction to silence gene expression. Ago1, Argonaute 1; Ago2, Argonaute 2; shRNA, short hairpin RNA; RISC, RNA induced silencing complex; RITS, RNA-induced transcriptional silencing complex; TRBP, trans-activating response RNA-binding protein; TNRC6, trinucleotide repeat containing six proteins.

to the enormous diversity of the genome, a multiplexed approach would be necessary to provide adequate coverage across HIV subtypes and strains. Additionally, as its silencing effects are only transient, PTGS would require either (1) frequent siRNA administration to an infected individual, thus rendering it a recurring treatment and not a cure, or (2) provision of a self-sustaining system. This would involve viral vector delivery of a plasmid that can constitutively express target siRNAs. This may be in the form of short hairpin (sh)RNAs that are exported to the cytoplasm and processed into the desired siRNA. The greatest pitfall however, is that PTGS predominately functions in the cytoplasm, targeting mRNA from an actively transcribing provirus. As such, it cannot overcome the selective pressures driving HIV-1 mutation. Rather, this process allows the virus to rapidly transcribe escape variants [50]. From point mutations and deletions that disrupt target specificity, to the generation of alternative secondary structures to prevent RISC accessibility [51], HIV-1 can rapidly circumvent a single PTGS therapeutic. Similar to ART, current PTGS therapeutics are having to be combined, to simultaneously target multiple HIV proteins and/or to target host targets, such as CCR5, to overcome the generation of resistance mutations [52].

3.2.2.1. RNA-directed latency inducing agents

In comparison, TGS can be considered the nucleic arm of RNAi. It offers the highly specific targeting of the integrated HIV provirus. Still controversial in mammals, this pathway begins in the cytoplasm where siRNA associate with Argonaute 1 protein (Ago1). These two components are trafficked to the nucleus [53] and recruit other proteins to form the RNA-induced transcriptional silencing (RITS) complex. The RITS protein components have been identified in *S. pombe* yeast and include Ago1, the GW protein, Tas3, and chromodomain protein 1 (Chp1) [54], however while Ago1 is present in mammalian cells, Tas3 and Chp1 homologues have not yet been identified. Although this complex can be considered as the equivalent of RISC from PTGS, it is not identical, due to the different functional requirements and distinct protein components. Via siRNA sequence complementarity, RITS identifies the target locus and induces chromatin compaction through epigenetic modifications, such as histone methylation [55]. By rendering it structurally inaccessible to transcriptional machinery, TGS can lock the virus in a latent state.

Like PTGS, TGS is capable of significantly suppressing HIV-1 production and is highly sequence specific, with minimal off-target effects and interferon mediated immune responses or defence mechanisms, dependent on the specific sequence targeted [56]. A single nucleotide mismatch between the siRNA and its target could be sufficient to disrupt silencing. Hence, conserved regions of the provirus must be carefully selected and a multiplexed approach may be necessary. TGS also offers several advantages over its cytoplasmic counterpart. By preventing the provirus from actively transcribing, it can silence HIV-1 prior to the generation of escape variants. Additionally, due to the heritable nature of the heterochromatin marks, daughter cells exhibit the same suppressive phenotype [57].

Our laboratory has described two siRNA sequences capable of inducing potent TGS in HIV-infected cells. The first siRNA, termed siPromA, was identified in 2005 and has been extensively characterised as inducing highly-sequence specific TGS via epigenetic repressive mechanisms [53, 55, 56, 58–60]. The siPromA sequence targets NF-κB tandem repeat motif, which is unique to the virus and is not homologous to any host cell NF-κB motifs. This is important as NF-κB is an important transcription factor for multiple cell signalling pathways. A second siRNA, termed si143, has recently been shown to also induce TGS and targets the COUP-TF and AP-1 transcription factor sites upstream of the siPromA target sequence [61]. When combined, these two siRNAs provide enhanced suppression and enforcement of latency through multiple epigenetic modifications. We have shown up to 1000-fold suppression of virus transcription following a single transfection of siPromA or si143 for up to 15 days in various HIV-infected cell cultures, including HeLa T4+ cells and Hut78 cells. Further, in MOLT-4 cells carrying shRNA expressing siPromA, we reported virus transcription was suppressed for over 1 year [60]. Specific epigenetic modifications in HIV cultures suppressed by siPromA or si143 have been investigated using ChIP assays and included enrichment of histone methylation on the N-terminal histone tail (such as HeK27me3, H3K9me2) and decreased acetylation (such as H3K9) [61]. We have also demonstrated effective *in vivo* virus suppression using a humanised mouse model of acute HIV in (NOD)/SCID/Janus kinase 3 (NOJ) knockout mice infected with

HIV-$1_{JR\text{-}FL}$. In human PBMCs that were stably transduced with shPromA delivered by a lentivirus vector and transplanted into the NOJ mice, followed by immune reconstitution, mice were protected from HIV-1 challenge, with significantly decreased plasma viral loads and normal CD4:CD8 T cell ratios, compared to control group treated with cells transduced with an inactive siRNA sequence carrying three mismatches (shPromA-M2) [58]. We anticipate, much like combined ART, that a multiplexed approach of combining TGS-inducing siRNAs will be necessary to provide sufficient control across a wide range of HIV subtypes and strains.

The Chattopadhyay laboratory has also reported a TGS-inducing siRNA sequence specifically targeting the HIV-1 subtype C NF-κB triple repeat motif, termed S4-siRNA. They demonstrated S4-siRNA induced TGS in a TZM-bl cell line and *ex vivo* human PBMCs transfected with S4-siRNA and infected with various subtype C viruses, as determined by measuring viral RNA levels [62]. Further, ChIP assay confirmed the enrichment of epigenetic repressive marks using histone methylation markers, H3K27me3 and H3K9me2. This siRNA may have potential as an RNA therapeutic, since HIV-1 subtype C is prevalent in approximately half of the people living with HIV globally.

3.2.2.2. RNA-aptamer silencing

The Morris laboratory has also described a TGS-inducing siRNA, termed, LTR362, which also targets the NF-κB tandem repeat motif [63] and overlaps with 8 bp of the siPromA sequence. This RNA therapeutic has recently been further developed with the addition of a delivery aptamer designed to the HIV-1 glycoprotein termed gp120 A-1 and multiplexing with PTGS-inducing siRNAs targeting Tat and Rev. [64], designed by the Rossi laboratory. They showed the LTR362 RNA localised to the nucleus of an HIV-infected T lyphoblastoid CEM cell line and primary human CD4+ T cells. Virus suppression showed a 10-fold reduction of viral p24 levels compared to control cultures at 12 days post-infection. This potential dual therapeutic was assessed *in vivo* using an HIV-1 infected humanised NOD/SCID/IL2 $r\gamma^{null}$ mouse model and demonstrated suppressed virus infection and protected CD4+ T cell levels in viremic mice. However, the mechanism of virus suppression was determined to be PTGS, due to the lack of the CpG methylation, an epigenetic silencing mark, at the 5′LTR. Investigation of histone methylation may prove some involvement of TGS, however the study currently indicates that while cell-type specific aptamer delivery of TGS-inducing siRNA functions *in vitro*, the *in vivo* silencing effect will require significant optimising to achieve robust epigenetic modifications [64].

4. Successful gene therapy treatment of HIV-1: the "Berlin patient"

The first person cured of HIV-1 was Timothy Ray Brown, also known as the 'Berlin patient', who still today remains to be the only person to be cured of HIV-1. Diagnosed with HIV at the age of 29, the patient commenced ART [65], but then presented with acute myeloid leukaemia at the age of 40. At that stage the patient's HIV was controlled with ART and classified as stage A2; asymptomatic with a CD4+ T-cell count of 415 cells/μL [66]. ART interruption during the first initial treatment showed viral rebound, therefore ART was resumed and no further treatment was required until an acute myeloid leukaemia relapse 7 month after initial treatment [66]. The patient then received an allogeneic haematopoietic stem-cell transplantation (HSCT)

[65, 66]. HSCT was already shown to be feasible in HIV positive patients, but it was also known that HSCT alone was insufficient to eliminate HIV [67]. For many patients finding an HLA-matched stem-cell donor is a significant challenge, however a suitable match was identified for the Berlin patient and subsequent screens for possible donors with the homozygous CCR5-delta32 (CCR5Δ32/Δ32) allele were performed [65, 66]. High resistance against HIV infection has been reported for individuals who are homozygous for the CCR5-delta32 deletion [68, 69]. HIV requires CD4 and typically either CCR5 (or CXCR4) for cell entry, making it a promising candidate for intervention [69]. Unlike CD4 and CXCR4, the absence of CCR5 is not obviously deleterious for modified cells [69]. Therefore the approach to use CCR5-delta32 stem-cells for HSCT of HIV infected patients was pursued, as earlier described by Chow et al., in 2001 [70]. Using this treatment approach an HLA-matched stem-cell donor with the homozygous CCR5-delta32 allele was identified [66].

The patient ceased ART medication on the day prior to the HSCT procedure, which was successful with complete chimerism achieved and only grade I graft-versus-host disease (GvHD) as serious complications [66]. HIV infection was analysed by RNA and DNA-PCR and remained undetectable in peripheral blood and bone marrow, as well as in the rectal mucosa [66]. Analysis of macrophages in the intestinal mucosa found they were still expressing CCR5, indicating that 159 days post-HSCT these long-lasting cells were not yet replaced by the new immune system [66]. The CD4+ T-cell count in peripheral blood stayed at a low level of less than 300 cells/μL after the first HSCT until leukaemia relapsed on day 332 after HSCT [66, 71]. Following a total body irradiation, the patient received a second HSCT from the same CCR5Δ32/Δ32 donor [66, 71]. Fortunately, after the second transplantation the HIV load remained undetectable for the following years in peripheral blood, bone marrow and tissue biopsies, including gut and brain [66, 71]. CCR5-expressing macrophages in the gut became undetectable over the years and the peripheral CD4+ T-cell count increased greatly within the first 6 month after the second HSCT, to over 400 cells/μL [71]. While the treatment was successful in inducing remission from the acute myeloid leukaemia, recovery from the second HSCT was slow, with a long period of infections, GvHD reactions in the liver and a period of fever, dizziness and delirium [65, 71]. The patient experienced loss of short-term memory, was almost paralysed and had to learn to walk again [65, 71].

As a milestone in HIV cure research, there is the question if this is a one-time wonder cure or if it is reproducible? In 2014, Hutter et al. assessed six more cases of patients with HIV-1 receiving an allogenic CCR5Δ32/Δ32 HSCT [72]. Five of those patients died within the first 4 months due to relapse, GvHD or infection [72]. The only patient surviving for 12 months experienced a rebound of CXCR4-tropic HIV-1 rapidly after the transplantation and died from a relapse of cancer [72]. This shows the difficulties of HSCT in HIV infected patients and the importance for careful selection of donor to recipient, as well as considering the continuance of ART to prevent CXCR4-tropic HIV-1 from rebounding until the new immune system has become more established [72]. In light of these attempts to replicate the successful treatment of Timothy Ray Brown, it should be noted that he was in fact Δ32 heterozygous prior to his HSCT, which likely provided him an advantage in relation to providing protection via Δ32 expression after transplantation.

The mechanisms of Berlin patient HIV cure are currently being investigated and pose an interesting question-is it a functional or sterilising cure? To start to answer this question, we will likely only be able to use the information currently available, as ongoing updates on this case may be limited due to the patient recently commencing pre-exposure prophylaxis (PrEP) in order to prevent contracting HIV a second time. Firstly, the patient had ceased taking ART for >4 years without experiencing viral rebound, secondly, the viral DNA level was below detection limit in the periphery and in tissue biopsies, and thirdly, the patient showed a decrease in anti-HIV antibodies, all indicating a lack of virus replication, which makes it possible to conclude that the patient is functionally cured of HIV [66, 71]. The principle of a sterilising cure is the complete eradication of a pathogen out of the human body. This would therefore mean that every single cell previously infected and therefore carrying the HIV-1 genome would need to be replaced by new donor-derived cells to completely eradicate HIV from the body. All tests for proviral DNA until now, showed no detectable HIV-DNA and Timothy Ray Brown remained without viral rebound for 4 years, indicating the possibility that even the long-lasting memory immune cells were replaced by cells derived from the donor. This could lead to the interpretation that it was in fact a sterilising cure. That being said it is important to take into account the current limits of detection and the fact every single cell in his body cannot be analysed. Further similar results were found in two other patients who did eventually rebound. Therefore, one cannot be definitive in whether the cure is functional or completely sterilising. Regardless of whether the final conclusion is potentially a sterilising cure, it was derived from a functional cure approach.

5. Genome editing

The ability to engineer specific changes in the genome of an organism has developed rapidly over the last 10 years. The technology of gene editing relies on nucleases, scissor-like enzymes, with the ability to cut genomic DNA in a highly specific manner. This process results in additions, deletions or alterations at the targeted site of the genome. There are two pathways that can achieve double stranded breaks (DSB) in DNA; (i) nonhomologous end joining (NHEJ) repair pathway, where deletions or insertions in the target gene result in gene disruption *e.g.* CCR5, or (ii) the homologous recombination or homology-directed repair (HDR) pathway, in which DNA sequences are introduced into the genome using a homologous DNA template. The HDR pathway is more precise, with limited off-target genome effects, due to more control over the integration site, copy number and expression of the DNA sequence [73]. Some examples of gene editing technologies include zinc finger nuclease (ZFN), transcription activator-like nucleases (TALENS), clustered regularly interspaced short palindromic repeats and CRISPR-associated protein 9 (CRISPR/Cas9). Examples of specific gene editing technologies that have been explored in the context of HIV treatment are described below.

5.1. Zinc finger nucleases (ZFN)

ZFNs are a combination of zinc-finger proteins, which have DNA recognition specificity, and the nuclease activity of the cleavage domain of restriction enzyme, *Fok*I. The most advanced ZFN pair targets the CCR5 host gene and HIV-1 co-receptor [74]. Preclinical studies in a mouse model, where mice received CD3/CD28-activated primary CD4+ T cells treated with the ZFN delivered in a chimeric adenoviral vector, Ad5/F35, showed anti-HIV efficacy, with disruption of 40–60% of all CCR5 alleles and 33% disruption of both CCR5 alleles [74]. Following the successful pre-clinical data, the ZFN progressed to phase I clinical studies and the first-in-human gene editing HIV treatment trial (#NCT00842634) commenced in 2009.

The primary outcome of this study investigated the safety of ZFN modification of autologous CD4+ T cells being delivered to HIV positive individuals [75]. A secondary outcome measured immune reconstitution and HIV resistance. Twelve ART-treated patients with undetectable viral loads were enrolled in two cohorts dependent on CD4+ T cell count; cohort 1 included patients with CD4+ T cell count >450/mm^3, the median being 662/mm^3, and cohort 2 was patients with lower CD4+ T cells counts between 200 and 500/mm^3, the median being 272/mm^3 [75]. Patients received one infusion containing 5x10^7 autologous CD4+ T cells that were ZFN-modified. The infusion of ZFN-treated cells was deemed safe, with one serious adverse event reported that was infusion-related. All patients demonstrated engraftment, with the ZFN-modified cells being present for up to ≥42 months following infusion and showed expected characteristics. At 4 weeks post-infusion, cohort 1 ceased taking ART in a 12 week analytical treatment interruption (ATI), resulting in four out of six patients with detectable viral loads at 2–4 weeks post-ART cessation [75]. One of the six patients experienced a delayed increase in viral load at week 6, but was still below the viral set point [75]. This patient was later determined to be heterozygous for CCR5Δ32, suggesting that this genotype enhanced the ZFN treatment effect.

The successful modification of CD34+ HPSCs was also shown using the same ZFN pair [76]. This has been further optimised to achieve HDR-induced gene modifications using an adeno-associated virus vector (AAV) serotype 6 and electroporation to deliver nuclease mRNA to both primary CD4+ T cells and HPSCs [77], achieving between 8 and 60% and 15–40% CCR5 editing, respectively. Currently, there is no *in vivo* method that can effectively deliver nucleases to cells infected with HIV, and this will require further characterisation of the HIV sanctuary sites and identification of latent cell markers to allow specific targeting of cells that comprise the virus reservoir.

The generation of off-target genome modification is also a concern for the clinical application of ZFNs. This is exemplified by the off-target effect reported for the highly related CCR2 gene which was disrupted in 5.39% of ZFN-modified CD4+ T cells that were targeting CCR5 and decreased CCR5 expression by 36% [74]. Optimisation of the CCR5 ZFN would be required if this off-target effect was determined to be deleterious.

5.2. CRISPR/Cas9

The development of therapeutics using CRISPR/Cas9 technology has rapidly intensified over the last decade. The system is based on a short guide RNA (gRNA) that targets a specific DNA sequence and the Cas9 endonuclease, which then cleaves the double stranded DNA. Mutations, either deletions or insertions, are introduced into the target sequence following DNA repair by the NHEJ repair pathway. Similar to ART, HIV has been shown to develop virus escape mutations when only a single gRNA is utilised and requires multiple gRNAs to prevent the emergences of virus resistance [78, 79]. Multiple studies have reported HIV-1 inactivation using this gene editing platform with dual gRNAs, via mutation at either target sites or complete excision of the virus sequence between the two target sites [80–83].

Although CRISPR technology has proven successful in inactivating HIV-1, like the ZFN system, successful delivery to all cells of the latent reservoir will be challenging without a known latency marker.

The CRISPR/Cas9 platform has recently been adapted to activate HIV transcription, akin to the "shock and kill" approach. This involves a mutation in the Cas9 catalytic domain which results in deactivated Cas9 (dCas9). The dCas9 can then be coupled to a strong transcription activation domain (AD) and targeted to the HIV-1 LTR can induce transcriptional activation via recruitment of transcription and chromatin modifying factors. One example of the dCas9-AD system is dCas9-VP64, which contains multiple copies of the herpes simplex virus (HSV) VP16-drived minimal AD and has been shown to activate HIV-1 promoter-driven gene expression. Interestingly, the most promising gRNA target in the HIV-1 5′LTR is single guide (sg)362F [84] and similar to the siPromA sequence described in the "block and lock" approach, targets the NF-κB binding motif.

6. Delivery

6.1. *Ex vivo* delivery by lentiviral vectors

Delivery of gene therapy to a specific target cell is another current challenge for an HIV cure. Viral vectors have become a regular method by which to deliver therapeutic genes and constructs [85]. There are multiple viable types of viral vectors that have been proven to be safe, relatively easy to construct and modify, and in the case of lentiviral vectors, these have the potential to transduce cells in a non-proliferative state [86]. Although the latter feature does not extend to non-proliferative leukocytes, due the presence of lentiviral restriction factors at and below the membrane.

One significant obstacle to the effective delivery of sufficient quantities viral vector is the ability to transduce sufficient quantities of target cells. To overcome this, apheresis is performed in order to concentrate the desired cells. Currently, gene therapy protocols for HIV first require the isolation of the desired cells to be modified, typically following apheresis [85]. Apheresis is the process of removing mononuclear cells from blood and returning neutrophils, platelets, plasma and red blood cells to the donor. This process is performed in order to collect more of the desired cells of the blood than could be separated from a unit of whole blood of ~550 mL. While CD4+ T cells are the main target for HIV infection, other cells such as dendritic cells, macrophages, monocytes and to a lesser extent, haematopoietic stem cells (HSC) have been found to be susceptible to HIV infection [87–89]. It is known that if HSC are transduced, or modified in any way, then a wide range of subsequent immune cells including macrophages, dendritic cells, CD4+ T cells and NK cells will carry that modification [90]. While transduction of CD4+ T cells will result in only CD4+ T cells being modified, the approach of transducing HSC provides protection from HIV to a broader range of cell-types, making it a highly desirable target for treatment/modification. Once a large volume of cells has been collected over several hours, they can then be transduced with the desired viral vector and reintroduced to the individual where the cells will migrate back to peripheral blood, lymph nodes, and bone marrow. This delivery method has been used in dozens of clinical trials and has become a widely accepted method for delivering viral vectors to large numbers of cells, in particular to HSC in the bone marrow [85]. The *ex vivo* gene therapy process is depicted in **Figure 4**.

As HSC predominantly reside in the bone marrow, in order to increase the quantity of HSC in peripheral blood, it is common to use granulocyte colony stimulating factor (G-CSF) as a mobilising agent to encourage recirculation of HSC. This causes cells to migrate from the bone marrow and lymph tissue into the peripheral blood. The use of G-CSF or other stimulating factors is essential when HSC are to be transduced with the therapeutic gene/vector, with various trials showing that HSC cell counts in peripheral blood increase 20–50-fold over the course of G-CSF administration [91–93]. To aid with re-engraftment of HSC back into the bone marrow after transduction, a technique known as myeloablation has been utilised in some clinical trials prior to the reintroduction of HSC via infusion, in order to provide an immunological niche and improve engraftment of the gene-containing cells [94]. This procedure involves the eradication of resident HSC, thereby reducing the population of non-transduced cells, and creating more space for the transduced cell population to reconstitute the bone marrow. A delay of the presence of newly 'protected CD4+ T cell' population would

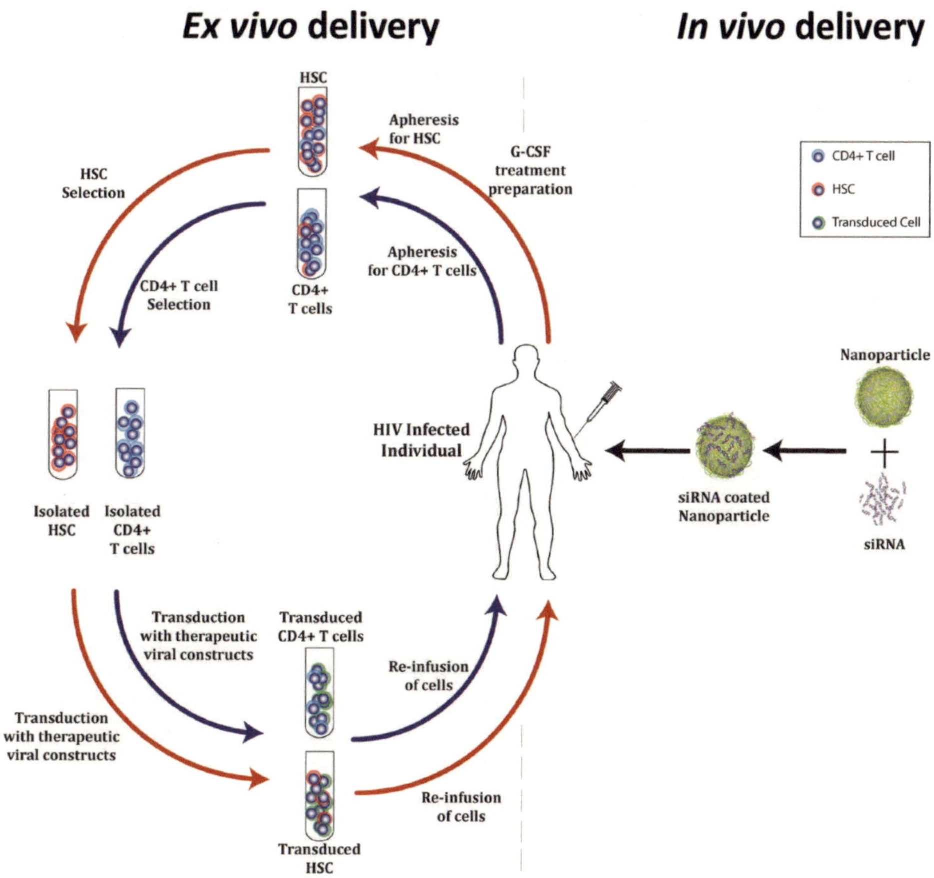

Figure 4. Gene therapy delivery strategies; *ex vivo* lentivirus transduction of isolated patient haematoepoetic stem cells (HSC) and/or CD4+ T cells to deliver the gene modification versus systemic, *in vivo* delivery of the gene therapy directly to the patient, which requires a cell specific moiety to ensure targeted cell delivery.

be expected due to the required production of cells, thus delaying the effect of the therapeutic gene(s). Production of new CD4+ T lymphocytes from the thymus has been predicted to be at a rate of approximately 1.65 cells/μL of blood/day due to thymic function [95]. The resulting in the production of a stable population of protected cells would be expected to gradually create a positive impact on CD4+ T cell number and help suppress viral load.

While the modification of HSC has the benefit of long-lasting and broad-spectrum protection via the differentiation of stem cells, this approach still lacks the immediate benefit of targeting the existing CD4+ T cells population. The use of CD4+ T cells as a target for HIV gene therapy has been explored and assessed in several studies. Isolation and modification of CD4+ T cells is relatively simple, as they largely populate and consistently traffic through peripheral blood. Accordingly, no stimulatory factors (such as G-CSF) are required to mobilise them prior to collection. This method has the benefits of providing an immediate benefit via the reintroduction of a protected population of the primary target cells for HIV infection [96]. This has been performed and shown to be both safe in treatment, and effective in delivery of the therapeutic gene [96, 97].

Lentiviral vectors are being increasingly used in clinical trials to treat a variety of diseases ranging from cancers, to genetic diseases such as haemophilia and sickle cell anaemia, as well as several trials treating HIV. The largest such trial in HIV gene therapy demonstrating the safety of lentiviral vectors was the Phase II trial whereby a Tat/Vpr specific anti-HIV ribozyme (OZ1) or placebo was delivered in autologous CD34+ haematopoietic progenitor cells. The trial involved 74 patients where there were no adverse events related to the vectors or infusion process [98].

As outlined above, present gene therapy efforts to target HIV are primarily defensive in approach, as they encode future HIV resistance and may not influence the HIV reservoir in the short-term. Given the success of CAR T cell therapy in various cancer trials, many investigators are now multiplexing HIV resistance alongside a CAR construct that can target HIV. As cellular markers for the HIV reservoir are often shared in various leukocyte niches, the equivalent to the anti-CD19 approach used in B cell leukaemia has yet to be determined. Rather, investigators have now turned to potent broadly neutralising antibodies, which have been screened and cloned from various HIV positive patients and target HIV envelope. In this setting, several pre-clinical studies are underway in non-human primates in the laboratories of Kiem and Jerome, where resistance afforded by C46 and shRNA is complexed with one of several CAR modules that incorporates the single variable change of well characterised broadly neutralising antibodies [99].

In contrast, work led by the Berger laboratory has taken a similar but different approach to CAR T cell development. Rather than incorporating a neutralising antibody, they have complexed the first Ig-Like domains of CD4 with the serum mannose binding lectin [100]. This approach enables global recognition of HIV envelope, as it engages the CD4 binding site and also the abundant glycosylation sites that decorate the antigenic silent face of HIV Env. In the CAR T cell context, CD8+ T cells are generated alongside HIV resistant CD4+ T cells to mediate attack on the HIV reservoir. The only problem with the latter approach is that the major HIV reservoir *in vivo* resides in the germinal centers of secondary lymphoid tissue and actively excludes CD8+ T cells, given they lack the germinal homing receptor CXCR5. Therefore, whilst CD4+ T cells may transverse the germinal center, CD8+ T cells will not.

To overcome this lack of secondary lymphoid targeting of CAR CD8+ T cells, the Skinner laboratory has recently developed a hybrid CAR construct that encompasses not only HIV targeting, but also the CXCR5 receptor [101]. In theory, this enables CD8+ T cells not only to target the HIV reservoir, but also transverse the site where the reservoir is located.

6.1.1. *Cal-1 lentiviral vector*

One vector of note that has been extensively studied is the Cal-1 vector, which uses both the maC46 fusion inhibitor and shRNA-CCR5. This construct has been extensively studied, consistently showing therapeutic benefits *in vitro*. Additionally, this construct has also shown its enhanced efficacy when compared against individual genes, as the effect is induced by the use of two therapeutic targets [102]. This has not only led to stronger protection from HIV infection, but also is likely to result in reduced risk of mutation resistance [102]. This has been examined in mouse studies and non-human primates, where it has shown safety, high levels of engraftment (including in CD34+ cells), and a selective growth advantage [102–105].

The Cal-1 therapeutic construct is currently undergoing Phase I/II clinical trials [106]. The study involves 12 HIV positive patients, which have undergone transduction of both HSC and CD4+ T cells with a lentiviral vector carrying both the shRNA-CCR5 and C46 fusion inhibitor. The patients were divided into 3 equal groups, group 1 received no busulfan pre-conditioning, group 2 received 4 mg/kg busulfan, and group 3 received 2 doses to a total of 6 mg/kg busulfan conditioning. This study is currently ongoing but will provide important data on the optimised conditioning treatment to guide future treatment studies.

6.1.2. *Limitations of lentiviral vector delivery*

Whilst we now have therapeutic approaches that can focus our efforts on a HIV cure, delivery of these components still presents a barrier. Lentiviral vectors have proven to be extremely useful in providing delivery of therapeutic genes, although there are still limitations. As mentioned, cells can only be modified *ex vivo*, thus requiring apheresis. Additionally, in the case of HIV, as ART will prevent uptake of the lentiviral vector, patients must first stop ART, thus raising various health concerns and ethical obstacles. Furthermore, current approved lentiviral platforms can only transduce T cells that are activated, as this over comes lentiviral restrictions at the membrane and underneath the membrane. The sum of these problems significantly increases the cost of the clinical approach. In the setting of CAR-T cells the estimates for treatment of refractory B cell leukaemia is approximately $US400,000. Given this substantial cost, the accessibility of this type of therapeutic intervention is low. Thus, efforts are underway that will improve the process of this gene delivery pipeline. For instance, lentiviral vectors could be developed to target fresh leukocyte populations *ex vivo*, obviating the need for large scale apheresis. Additionally, lentiviral vectors could be modified to target leukocyte subsets, so the cells with the greatest stem-like attributes are re-infused and not diluted with cells that may not proceed down the differentiation pathway. This could potentially include a sub-population of resting T cells (*e.g.* Stem T cells) being isolated, genetically modified and re-infused in a manner that may not require apheresis. However, whether re-infusion of a smaller population of stem T cell would result in the same outcome that maybe achieved with a large population of bulk T cells obtained by leukopheresis needs to be thoroughly investigated.

6.2. *In vivo* delivery by nanoparticles

The *ex vivo* delivery of an HIV gene therapy treatment will only be achievable in developed countries with the appropriate resources to facilitate the approach and this will not be feasible in countries which currently have the largest burden of HIV, such as sub-Saharan Africa. We and others are working on an alternate and highly relevant systemic, *in vivo* approach, which may ultimately be accessible to all. This approach utilises nanotechnology to deliver the HIV therapeutic to target cells, ideally those of the latent reservoir. According to the Recommendation of the European Commission in 2011 the currently accepted definition of a nanoparticle (NP) is a particle where one or more external dimensions is in the size range of 1 to 100 nm [107]. However, larger particles with sizes up 1000 and 2000 nanometres are commonly referred to as 'nano', especially since for medical purposes the size range of ≤100 nm is not always practical, as a larger surface can carry more drug on a single particle [108, 109]. However, to be able to be used in the human body, NPs must be biocompatible and without cytotoxic side effects [108, 109].

Concentrating on HIV drug delivery, NPs have the unique feature of being able to absorb and carry other compounds on their relatively large functional surface [109]. Using NPs as delivery agents has the potential advantages of highly specific and controlled drug delivery to a targeted tissue or cell, such as those of the latent reservoir, keeping non-target organs and cells free of the drug, thereby reducing toxicity. Further, by releasing the drug in a controlled manner at a predetermined rate, achieved through changes in the physiological environment like pH, temperature or enzymatic activity, the resulting therapeutic efficacy can be increased [108–110]. Importantly, nano-based delivery systems have been shown to transport therapeutics across the blood-brain barrier, which is highly relevant for treating neuro-degenerative diseases and specifically the HIV reservoir in the central nervous system [111]. Prior to use of NPs in humans, the following basic prerequisites need to be known: drug incorporation and release, formulation stability and shelf life, biocompatibility, biodistribution and targeting, potential toxicities as well as functionality [109]. Another consideration are the possible adverse effects of residual material after drug delivery, therefore biodegradable NPs with a limited life span are optimal [109].

There are many types of NPs reported as delivery vehicles for HIV therapeutics, such as liposomes, micelles, polymer capsules, inorganic gold particles and dendrimers [112]. The number of different formulations of NPs being explored for HIV and other diseases is steadily increasing and a focused review on nanoparticle systems is provided by Pelaz et al. [112]. An example of the *in vivo* gene therapy process is depicted in **Figure 4**.

In the case of HIV, NPs have been used to deliver antiretroviral drugs or anti-HIV therapeutics, such as siRNAs. Inorganic gold particles delivering antiretrovirals have progressed through to *in vivo* delivery in mouse models, as have poly(amidoamine) PAMAM dendrimers and RNA-aptamer conjugates (as previously describes in Section 3.2.2.2), that deliver a combination of anti-HIV siRNAs. The gold particles and PAMAM dendrimer nano-platforms will be discussed below to highlight the challenges of targeting the HIV latent reservoir.

The NP platforms delivering an antiretroviral drug were comprised of inorganic gold nanoparticles particles (AuNPs) ~2–10 nanometers in diameter and were conjugated with an HIV integrase inhibitor, raltegravir [113]. Modification of raltegravir was necessary to link the inhibitor to the gold nanoparticle and involved incorporation of a thiol group to generate thiolated raltegravir. Cellular uptake and toxicity of AuNps was assessed in three different cell types; PBMCs, macrophages and HBMECs and confocal microscopy showed AuNPs inside all three cell types 24 hours post-delivery [113]. No toxicity was observed between 24 and 72 hours post-delivery. Importantly, the study investigated *in vivo* delivery of AuNPs and reported the presence of AuNPs in multiple sites, with the highest to lowest levels observed in spleen, liver, kidney, tail, heart, blood, lungs, muscle and brain of BALB mice 24 hours post-delivery [113]. Accumulation of AuNPs in the spleen and liver was attributed to reticuloendothelial system clearance, which is the bodies first line of defence for any *in vivo* delivered therapy. The lack of a specific marker for the latent reservoir is an ongoing challenge for targeting cells which harbour integrated HIV DNA and have the potential to reactivate and produce productive virus. Although this approach does successfully penetrate some cells of the latent reservoir, *i.e.* lymphocytes and macrophages, and to a modest degree cells in the brain, it is not a targeted approach and will most likely need further development of functional groups to penetrate the majority of cells of the latent reservoir. Due to the rarity of cells harbouring latent provirus, which is estimated to be 1 in every 10^6 cells, targeting these cells is the current challenge for an HIV cure.

The cationic PAMAM dendrimer NP system is comprised of highly branched, chemical polymers with cationic primary amine groups on a spherical surface that form stable, uniform nanoscale complexes. The PAMAM dendrimer interacts electrostatically with negatively charged dicer substrate siRNAs (dsiRNAs). The combination of anti-HIV siRNAs in this study included tat/rev, as well as the siRNAs targeting the CD4 and TNP03 genes [114]. In this study, humanised Rag2^{-}/$^{-}\gamma$c^{-}/$^{-}$ mice were generated and infected with HIV-1$_{NL4-3}$ 12 weeks following engraftment, then dendrimer-siRNA complexes were delivered via *i.v.* injection using equal amounts of all three siRNAs. Injections were continued weekly for 4 weeks. A significant decrease in HIV viral load by 3 logs relative to controls was reported and persisted up to 3 weeks post-treatment, however virus rebound was observed in the majority of animals after this time point [114], as is the standard response in patients following ART cessation. The study then investigated redosing of the dendrimer-siRNA complexes 3 months following the last administration and observed a further virus suppression which persisted for 3 weeks past the additional treatment. Assessment of mRNA levels of the three targeted genes (HIV tat/rev, CD4 and TNPO3) showed reductions in mRNA levels relative to the controls corresponded to the dosing schedule and confirmed sequence-specific and efficient gene silencing [114]. The main challenge with this approach is the need for continual treatment, or alternately the further development of a sustained-release approach. Further, whether this approach will be able to target very rare cells harbouring the latent reservoir remains to be investigated.

7. Conclusion

The field of HIV gene therapy is rapidly evolving, with development of both novel anti-HIV therapeutics and delivery systems to ensure cell specific targeting. While an *ex vivo* gene therapy approach for HIV is well on the path to patient translation, further targeting of the latent reservoir will be necessary to achieve a systemic, *in vivo* gene therapy approach. This will require identification of biomarker/s for latently-infected cells and novel ways to incorporate them into viral vectors and/or nanoparticle platforms. Once achieved, the next challenge will be the cost of treatment, which is becoming a driving factor in the context of HIV, as the global burden of HIV is predominantly in sub-Saharan Africa. The cost of *ex vivo* gene therapy approaches is prohibitive in developing countries and *in vivo* nanoparticle approaches, whilst more cost effective, do not yet achieve sustained virus remission. Further optimisation and refinement of current delivery systems is required to enable wide scale application of a functional HIV cure.

Acknowledgements

This work was supported by a National Health and Medical Research Council Project Grant APP1128012.

Conflict of interest

The authors declare no conflict of interest. GS, AK and CA hold patents for si/shRNA protection against HIV-1 and GS is an employee of Calimmune Inc./CSL.

Author details

Katherine Ognenovska[1], Vera Klemm[1], Scott Ledger[1], Stuart Turville[1], Geoff Symonds[2], Anthony D. Kelleher[1] and Chantelle L. Ahlenstiel[1*]

*Address all correspondence to: cahlenstiel@kirby.unsw.edu.au

1 Kirby Institute, UNSW, Sydney, NSW, Australia

2 Calimmune/CSL, Darlinghurst, NSW, Australia

References

[1] Global AIDS Update 2016. Available from: http://www.who.int/hiv/pub/arv/global-AIDS-update-2016_en.pdf?ua=1

[2] PrEPWatch. PrEPWatch - Country Updates - Track Global PrEP Use. 2018 March 27th, 2018. Available from: https://www.prepwatch.org/scaling-up/country-updates/

[3] Grant RM et al. Uptake of pre-exposure prophylaxis, sexual practices, and HIV incidence in men and transgender women who have sex with men: A cohort study. The Lancet Infectious Diseases. 2014;**14**(9):820-829

[4] Marrazzo JM et al. Tenofovir-based preexposure prophylaxis for HIV infection among African women. The New England Journal of Medicine. 2015;**372**(6):509-518

[5] Bavinton B, Grinsztejn B, Phanuphak N, Jin F, Zablotska I, et al. The Opposites Attract Study Group. HIV Treatment Prevents HIV Transmission in Male Serodiscordant Couples in Australia, Thailand and Brazil. IAS 2017, Paris, France, 2017; 2017: p. http://programme.ias2017.org/Abstract/Abstract/5469

[6] Bavinton BR et al. The opposites attract study of viral load, HIV treatment and HIV transmission in serodiscordant homosexual male couples: Design and methods. BMC Public Health. 2014;**14**:917

[7] Rodger AJ et al. Sexual activity without condoms and risk of HIV transmission in serodifferent couples when the HIV-positive partner is using suppressive antiretroviral therapy. JAMA. 2016;**316**(2):171-181

[8] Hiener B et al. Identification of genetically intact HIV-1 proviruses in specific CD4(+) T cells from effectively treated participants. Cell Reports. 2017;**21**(3):813-822

[9] Hufert FT et al. Germinal centre CD4+ T cells are an important site of HIV replication in vivo. AIDS. 1997;**11**(7):849-857

[10] Gomez C, Hope TJ. The ins and outs of HIV replication. Cellular Microbiology. 2005;**7**(5):621-626

[11] Jayappa KD, Ao Z, Yao X. The HIV-1 passage from cytoplasm to nucleus: The process involving a complex exchange between the components of HIV-1 and cellular machinery to access nucleus and successful integration. International Journal of Biochemistry and Molecular Biology. 2012;**3**(1):70-85

[12] Sundquist WI, Krausslich HG. HIV-1 assembly, budding, and maturation. Cold Spring Harbor Perspectives in Medicine. 2012;**2**(7):a006924

[13] Hubner W et al. Quantitative 3D video microscopy of HIV transfer across T cell virological synapses. Science. 2009;**323**(5922):1743-1747

[14] Dimitrov DS et al. Quantitation of human immunodeficiency virus type 1 infection kinetics. Journal of Virology. 1993;**67**(4):2182-2190

[15] Chiodi F et al. Isolation frequency of human immunodeficiency virus from cerebrospinal fluid and blood of patients with varying severity of HIV infection. AIDS Research and Human Retroviruses. 1988;**4**(5):351-358

[16] Ma M, Geiger JD, Nath A. Characterization of a novel binding site for the human immunodeficiency virus type 1 envelope protein gp120 on human fetal astrocytes. Journal of Virology. 1994;**68**(10):6824-6828

[17] Margolis DM. Mechanisms of HIV latency: An emerging picture of complexity. Current HIV/AIDS Reports. 2010;**7**(1):37-43

[18] Finzi D et al. Latent infection of CD4+ T cells provides a mechanism for lifelong persistence of HIV-1, even in patients on effective combination therapy. Nature Medicine. 1999;**5**(5):512-517

[19] Siliciano RF, Greene WC. HIV latency. Cold Spring Harbor Perspectives in Medicine. 2011;**1**(1):a007096

[20] Banga R et al. PD-1(+) and follicular helper T cells are responsible for persistent HIV-1 transcription in treated aviremic individuals. Nature Medicine. 2016;**22**(7):754-761

[21] Yukl SA et al. The distribution of HIV DNA and RNA in cell subsets differs in gut and blood of HIV-positive patients on ART: Implications for viral persistence. The Journal of Infectious Diseases. 2013;**208**(8):1212-1220

[22] Frauwirth KA, Thompson CB. Regulation of T lymphocyte metabolism. Journal of Immunology. 2004;**172**(8):4661-4665

[23] Liu JO. The yins of T cell activation. Science's STKE. 2005;**2005**(265):re1

[24] Perkins ND et al. A cooperative interaction between NF-kappa B and Sp1 is required for HIV-1 enhancer activation. The EMBO Journal. 1993;**12**(9):3551-3558

[25] Coiras M et al. Basal shuttle of NF-kappaB/I kappaB alpha in resting T lymphocytes regulates HIV-1 LTR dependent expression. Retrovirology. 2007;**4**:56

[26] Cron RQ et al. NFAT1 enhances HIV-1 gene expression in primary human CD4 T cells. Clinical Immunology. 2000;**94**(3):179-191

[27] Stellbrink HJ et al. Effects of interleukin-2 plus highly active antiretroviral therapy on HIV-1 replication and proviral DNA (COSMIC trial). AIDS. 2002;**16**(11):1479-1487

[28] Lafeuillade A et al. Pilot study of a combination of highly active antiretroviral therapy and cytokines to induce HIV-1 remission. Journal of Acquired Immune Deficiency Syndromes. 2001;**26**(1):44-55

[29] Sagot-Lerolle N et al. Prolonged valproic acid treatment does not reduce the size of latent HIV reservoir. AIDS. 2008;**22**(10):1125-1129

[30] Hording M et al. Lack of immunomodulating effect of disulfiram on HIV positive pa-tients. International Journal of Immunopharmacology. 1990;**12**(2):145-147

[31] Prins JM et al. Immuno-activation with anti-CD3 and recombinant human IL-2 in HIV-1-infected patients on potent antiretroviral therapy. AIDS. 1999;**13**(17):2405-2410

[32] Rasmussen TA et al. Panobinostat, a histone deacetylase inhibitor, for latent-virus reactivation in HIV-infected patients on suppressive antiretroviral therapy: A phase 1/2, single group, clinical trial. Lancet HIV. 2014;**1**(1):e13-e21

[33] Kim Y, Anderson JL, Lewin SR. Getting the "kill" into "shock and kill": Strategies to eliminate latent HIV. Cell Host & Microbe. 2018;**23**(1):14-26

[34] Wen J et al. Specific elimination of latently HIV-1 infected cells using HIV-1 protease-sensitive toxin nanocapsules. PLoS One. 2016;**11**(4):e0151572

[35] Mousseau G et al. An analog of the natural steroidal alkaloid cortistatin A potently suppresses Tat-dependent HIV transcription. Cell Host & Microbe. 2012;**12**(1):97-108

[36] Matzke MA et al. Reversible methylation and inactivation of marker genes in sequentially transformed tobacco plants. The EMBO Journal. 1989;**8**(3):643-649

[37] Mette MF et al. Transcriptional silencing and promoter methylation triggered by double-stranded RNA. The EMBO Journal. 2000;**19**(19):5194-5201

[38] Lippman Z et al. Distinct mechanisms determine transposon inheritance and methylation via small interfering RNA and histone modification. PLoS Biology. 2003;**1**(3):E67

[39] Fire A et al. Potent and specific genetic interference by double-stranded RNA in *Caenorhabditis elegans*. Nature. 1998;**391**(6669):806-811

[40] Martienssen RA, Zaratiegui M, Goto DB. RNA interference and heterochromatin in the fission yeast Schizosaccharomyces pombe. Trends in Genetics. 2005;**21**(8):450-456

[41] Filipowicz W et al. Post-transcriptional gene silencing by siRNAs and miRNAs. Current Opinion in Structural Biology. 2005;**15**(3):331-341

[42] Capodici J, Kariko K, Weissman D. Inhibition of HIV-1 infection by small interfering RNA-mediated RNA interference. Journal of Immunology. 2002;**169**(9):5196-5201

[43] Jacque JM, Triques K, Stevenson M. Modulation of HIV-1 replication by RNA interference. Nature. 2002;**418**(6896):435-438

[44] Boden D et al. Enhanced gene silencing of HIV-1 specific siRNA using microRNA designed hairpins. Nucleic Acids Research. 2004;**32**(3):1154-1158

[45] Lee MTM et al. Inhibition of human immunodeficiency virus type 1 replication in primary macrophages by using Tat- or CCR5-specific small interfering RNAs expressed from a lentivirus vector. Journal of Virology. 2003;**77**(22):11964-11972

[46] Lee NS et al. Expression of small interfering RNAs targeted against HIV-1 rev transcripts in human cells. Nature Biotechnology. 2002;**20**(5):500-505

[47] Semizarov D et al. Specificity of short interfering RNA determined through gene expression signatures. Proceedings of the National Academy of Sciences of the United States of America. 2003;**100**(11):6347-6352

[48] Reynolds A et al. Induction of the interferon response by siRNA is cell type- and duplex length-dependent. RNA. 2006;**12**(6):988-993

[49] Elbashir SM et al. Functional anatomy of siRNAs for mediating efficient RNAi in Drosophila melanogaster embryo lysate. The EMBO Journal. 2001;**20**(23):6877-6888

[50] Das AT et al. Human immunodeficiency virus type 1 escapes from RNA interference-mediated inhibition. Journal of Virology. 2004;**78**(5):2601-2605

[51] Westerhout EM et al. HIV-1 can escape from RNA interference by evolving an alternative structure in its RNA genome. Nucleic Acids Research. 2005;**33**(2):796-804

[52] ter Brake O et al. Lentiviral vector design for multiple shRNA expression and durable HIV-1 inhibition. Molecular Therapy. 2008;**16**(3):557-564

[53] Ahlenstiel CL et al. Direct evidence of nuclear Argonaute distribution during transcriptional silencing links the actin cytoskeleton to nuclear RNAi machinery in human cells. Nucleic Acids Research. 2012;**40**(4):1579-1595

[54] Verdel A et al. RNAi-mediated targeting of heterochromatin by the RITS complex. Science. 2004;**303**(5658):672-676

[55] Suzuki K et al. Closed chromatin architecture is induced by an RNA duplex targeting the HIV-1 promoter region. The Journal of Biological Chemistry. 2008;**283**(34):23353-23363

[56] Suzuki K et al. Transcriptional gene silencing of HIV-1 through promoter targeted RNA is highly specific. RNA Biology. 2011;**8**(6):1035-1046

[57] Probst AV, Dunleavy E, Almouzni G. Epigenetic inheritance during the cell cycle. Nature Reviews. Molecular Cell Biology. 2009;**10**(3):192-206

[58] Suzuki K et al. Promoter targeting shRNA suppresses HIV-1 infection in vivo through transcriptional gene silencing. Molecular Therapy--Nucleic Acids. 2013;**2**:e137

[59] Suzuki K et al. Prolonged transcriptional silencing and CpG methylation induced by siRNAs targeted to the HIV-1 promoter region. Journal of RNAi and Gene Silencing. 2005;**1**(2):66-78

[60] Yamagishi M et al. Retroviral delivery of promoter-targeted shRNA induces long-term silencing of HIV-1 transcription. Microbes and Infection. 2009;**11**(4):500-508

[61] Ahlenstiel C et al. Novel RNA duplex locks HIV-1 in a latent state via chromatin-mediated transcriptional silencing. Molecular Therapy--Nucleic Acids. 2015;**4**:e261

[62] Singh A et al. Long-term suppression of HIV-1C virus production in human peripheral blood mononuclear cells by LTR heterochromatization with a short double-stranded RNA. The Journal of Antimicrobial Chemotherapy. 2014;**69**(2):404-415

[63] Weinberg MS et al. The antisense strand of small interfering RNAs directs histone methylation and transcriptional gene silencing in human cells. RNA. 2006;**12**(2):256-262

[64] Zhou J et al. Receptor-targeted aptamer-siRNA conjugate-directed transcriptional regulation of HIV-1. Theranostics. 2018;**8**(6):1575-1590

[65] Brown TR. I am the Berlin patient: A personal reflection. AIDS Research and Human Retroviruses. 2015;**31**(1):2-3

[66] Hutter G et al. Long-term control of HIV by CCR5 Delta32/Delta32 stem-cell transplantation. The New England Journal of Medicine. 2009;**360**(7):692-698

[67] Hutter G, Zaia JA. Allogeneic haematopoietic stem cell transplantation in patients with human immunodeficiency virus: The experiences of more than 25 years. Clinical and Experimental Immunology. 2011;**163**(3):284-295

[68] Samson M et al. Resistance to HIV-1 infection in caucasian individuals bearing mutant alleles of the CCR-5 chemokine receptor gene. Nature. 1996;**382**(6593):722-725

[69] Alkhatib G. The biology of CCR5 and CXCR4. Current Opinion in HIV and AIDS. 2009;**4**(2):96-103

[70] Robert Chow DOR, Punzalan RR, Petz LD. Stem Cell Screening and Transplantation Therapy for HIV infection, in United States Patent Application Publication, U.S. Patent, Editor. 2001: US. p. 8

[71] Hutter G, Ganepola S. Eradication of HIV by transplantation of CCR5-deficient hematopoietic stem cells. ScientificWorldJournal. 2011;**11**:1068-1076

[72] Hutter G. More on shift of HIV tropism in stem-cell transplantation with CCR5 delta32/delta32 mutation. The New England Journal of Medicine. 2014;**371**(25):2437-2438

[73] Wang CX, Cannon PM. The clinical applications of genome editing in HIV. Blood. 2016;**127**(21):2546-2552

[74] Perez EE et al. Establishment of HIV-1 resistance in CD4+ T cells by genome editing using zinc-finger nucleases. Nature Biotechnology. 2008;**26**(7):808-816

[75] Tebas P et al. Gene editing of CCR5 in autologous CD4 T cells of persons infected with HIV. The New England Journal of Medicine. 2014;**370**(10):901-910

[76] Holt N et al. Human hematopoietic stem/progenitor cells modified by zinc-finger nucleases targeted to CCR5 control HIV-1 in vivo. Nature Biotechnology. 2010;**28**(8):839-847

[77] Wang J et al. Homology-driven genome editing in hematopoietic stem and progenitor cells using ZFN mRNA and AAV6 donors. Nature Biotechnology. 2015;**33**(12):1256-1263

[78] Wang G et al. A combinatorial CRISPR-Cas9 attack on HIV-1 DNA extinguishes all infectious provirus in infected T cell cultures. Cell Reports. 2016;**17**(11):2819-2826

[79] Wang Z et al. CRISPR/Cas9-derived mutations both inhibit HIV-1 replication and accelerate viral escape. Cell Reports. 2016;**15**(3):481-489

[80] Kaminski R et al. Excision of HIV-1 DNA by gene editing: A proof-of-concept in vivo study. Gene Therapy. 2016;**23**(8-9):690-695

[81] Kaminski R et al. Elimination of HIV-1 genomes from human T-lymphoid cells by CRISPR/Cas9 gene editing. Scientific Reports. 2016;**6**:22555

[82] Wang G et al. CRISPR-Cas9 can inhibit HIV-1 replication but NHEJ repair facilitates virus escape. Molecular Therapy. 2016;**24**(3):522-526

[83] Zhu W et al. The CRISPR/Cas9 system inactivates latent HIV-1 proviral DNA. Retrovirology. 2015;**12**:22

[84] Saayman SM et al. Potent and targeted activation of latent HIV-1 using the CRISPR/dCas9 activator complex. Molecular Therapy. 2016;**24**(3):488-498

[85] Symonds GP et al. The use of cell-delivered gene therapy for the treatment of HIV/AIDS. Immunologic Research. 2010;**48**(1-3):84-98

[86] Zufferey R et al. Self-inactivating lentivirus vector for safe and efficient in vivo gene delivery. Journal of Virology. 1998;**72**(12):9873-9880

[87] Carter CC et al. HIV-1 utilizes the CXCR4 chemokine receptor to infect multipotent hematopoietic stem and progenitor cells. Cell Host & Microbe. 2011;**9**(3):223-234

[88] Carter CC et al. HIV-1 infects multipotent progenitor cells causing cell death and establishing latent cellular reservoirs. Nature Medicine. 2010;**16**(4):446-451

[89] Stanley SK et al. CD34+ bone marrow cells are infected with HIV in a subset of seropositive individuals. Journal of Immunology. 1992;**149**(2):689-697

[90] Carter CA, Ehrlich LS. Cell biology of HIV-1 infection of macrophages. Annual Review of Microbiology. 2008;**62**:425-443

[91] Lane TA et al. Harvesting and enrichment of hematopoietic progenitor cells mobilized into the peripheral blood of normal donors by granulocyte-macrophage colony-stimulating factor (GM-CSF) or G-CSF: Potential role in allogeneic marrow transplantation. Blood. 1995;**85**(1):275-282

[92] Law P et al. Mobilization of peripheral blood progenitor cells for human immunodeficiency virus-infected individuals. Experimental Hematology. 1999;**27**(1):147-154

[93] Valgimigli M et al. Use of granulocyte-colony stimulating factor during acute myocardial infarction to enhance bone marrow stem cell mobilization in humans: Clinical and angiographic safety profile. European Heart Journal. 2005;**26**(18):1838-1845

[94] Strayer DS et al. Current status of gene therapy strategies to treat HIV/AIDS. Molecular Therapy. 2005;**11**(6):823-842

[95] Murray JM et al. Naive T cells are maintained by thymic output in early ages but by proliferation without phenotypic change after age twenty. Immunology and Cell Biology. 2003;**81**(6):487-495

[96] Levine BL et al. Gene transfer in humans using a conditionally replicating lentiviral vector. Proceedings of the National Academy of Sciences of the United States of America. 2006;**103**(46):17372-17377

[97] Brunstein CG et al. Infusion of ex vivo expanded T regulatory cells in adults transplanted with umbilical cord blood: Safety profile and detection kinetics. Blood. 2011; **117**(3):1061-1070

[98] Mitsuyasu RT et al. Phase 2 gene therapy trial of an anti-HIV ribozyme in autologous CD34+ cells. Nature Medicine. 2009;**15**(3):285-292

[99] Spragg C, De Silva Feelixge H, Jerome KR. Cell and gene therapy strategies to eradicate HIV reservoirs. Current Opinion in HIV and AIDS. 2016;**11**(4):442-449

[100] Ghanem MH et al. Bispecific chimeric antigen receptors targeting the CD4 binding site and high-mannose Glycans of gp120 optimized for anti-human immunodeficiency virus potency and breadth with minimal immunogenicity. Cytotherapy. 2018;**20**(3):407-419

[101] Haran KP et al. Simian immunodeficiency virus (SIV)-specific chimeric antigen receptor-T cells engineered to target B cell follicles and suppress SIV replication. Frontiers in Immunology. 2018;**9**:492

[102] Wolstein O et al. Preclinical safety and efficacy of an anti-HIV-1 lentiviral vector containing a short hairpin RNA to CCR5 and the C46 fusion inhibitor. Molecular Therapy - Methods & Clinical Development. 2014;**1**:11

[103] Burke BP et al. Engineering Cellular Resistance to HIV-1 Infection In Vivo Using a Dual Therapeutic Lentiviral Vector. Molecular Therapy--Nucleic Acids. 2015;**4**:e236

[104] Peterson CW et al. Multilineage polyclonal engraftment of Cal-1 gene-modified cells and in vivo selection after SHIV infection in a nonhuman primate model of AIDS. Molecular Therapy - Methods & Clinical Development. 2016;**3**:16007

[105] Ringpis GE et al. Engineering HIV-1-resistant T-cells from short-hairpin RNA-expressing hematopoietic stem/progenitor cells in humanized BLT mice. PLoS One. 2012;**7**(12):e53492

[106] Symonds G et al. Cell-delivered entry inhibitors for HIV-1: CCR5 downregulation and blocking virus/membrane fusion in defending the host cell population. AIDS Patient Care and STDs. 2016;**30**(12):545-550

[107] The European Commission, Commission Recommendation of 18 October 2011 on the definition of nanomaterial. 2011: Official Journal of the European Union

[108] Wilczewska AZ et al. Nanoparticles as drug delivery systems. Pharmacological Reports. 2012;**64**(5):1020-1037

[109] De Jong WH, Borm PJ. Drug delivery and nanoparticles: Applications and hazards. International Journal of Nanomedicine. 2008;**3**(2):133-149

[110] Rycroft T et al. Nanotoxicology and nanomedicine: Making development decisions in an evolving governance environment. Journal of Nanoparticle Research. 2018;**20**(2):52

[111] Saraiva C et al. Nanoparticle-mediated brain drug delivery: Overcoming blood–brain barrier to treat neurodegenerative diseases. Journal of Controlled Release. 2016;**235**:34-47

[112] Pelaz B et al. Diverse applications of nanomedicine. ACS Nano. 2017;**11**(3):2313-2381

[113] Garrido C et al. Gold nanoparticles to improve HIV drug delivery. Future Medicinal Chemistry. 2015;**7**(9):1097-1107

[114] Zhou J et al. Systemic administration of combinatorial dsiRNAs via nanoparticles efficiently suppresses HIV-1 infection in humanized mice. Molecular Therapy. 2011; **19**(12):2228-2238

Chapter 4

Functional Activation of Autologous Human Diabetic Stem Cells for Cell Therapy

Patrick L. Iversen, Francis W. Ruscetti,
Charles Garcia and Stephen H. Bartelmez

Additional information is available at the end of the chapter

http://dx.doi.org/10.5772/intechopen.79650

Abstract

Diabetic retinopathy (DR) is a common cause of vision loss and blindness. Healthy CD34+ stem cells are capable of homing to vascular lesions and facilitating vascular repair. However, many diabetic patients have dysfunctional CD34+ stem cells with no reparative potential. CD34+ dysfunction is corrected by transiently inhibiting endogenous transforming growth factor-β1 (TGF-β1) within the patient's own dysfunctional CD34+ stem cells using phosphorodiamidate morpholino oligomers (PMOs). Antisense TGF-β1-treated dysfunctional CD34+ stem cells are now functional, no longer require growth factor stimulation to evade apoptosis, and are stable at 37°C ex vivo for >5 days. We identified three markers of restored stem cell function: (1) upregulation of CXCR4 expression necessary for stem cell homing and adhesion, (2) SDF-1-mediated nitric oxide (NO) production required for cell mobility, and (3) restoration of the ability of CD34+ cells to migrate and repair vascular lesions. The antisense targets autocrine TGF-β expression, whereas neutralizing antibodies do not. The PMO antisense triggers a cascade of hematopoietic proliferation and differentiation that paracrine TGF-β cannot alter. We describe optimal PMO manipulation of CD34+ stem cells ex vivo for transplantation, screening multiple gene targets leading to the identification of TGF-β1, and a lead TGF-β1 inhibitor evaluated in clinical studies.

Keywords: diabetic retinopathy, stem cell therapy, transforming growth factor-β1 (TGF-β1), phosphorodiamidate morpholino oligomers (PMOs), transient antisense

1. Introduction

Hematopoietic stem cells (HSCs) are capable of self-replication and clonal expansion generating differentiated progenitors, which give rise to all blood cell lineages [1]. These cells co-express transforming growth factor-β (TGF-β) type I and type II receptors and one or more of the three isoforms of the TGF-β ligand as a latent complex [2]. The three TGF-β ligands qualitatively and quantitatively differ in the responses they elicit with TGF-β1, a multifunctional regulator of hematopoietic progenitors in vivo and in vitro, depending on cell differentiation, growth factors, ligand concentration, and cell–cell contacts [3]. Autocrine signaling by TGF-β1 plays a critical role in lineage-specific reconstitution [4] and enables non-canonical signaling involving mTOR, Ras, MAPK, PI3K, AKT, RhoA, and JNK [5]. TGF-β is an important part of the stromal microenvironment that regulates several niche cells, which in turn regulate HSC. Selective manipulation of endogenous TGF-β1 in HSC represents a therapeutic approach to transplantation to maintain, enhance, and restore tissue viability and organ function.

Transient inhibition of TGF-β1 in HSC accelerates the engraftment of long-term repopulating HSC (LTR-HSC), permits successful transplantation with as few as 60 LTR-HSCs to rescue mice from lethal irradiation, and promotes the survival of LTR-HSC in the absence of growth factors [6]. This permits LTR-HSC transplant without cell expansion ex vivo prior to transplant. TGF-β1 regulates LTR-HSC entry into the cell cycle at G0 [7]. Conditional knock-out of the TGF-β1 type II receptor in adult mice has increased stem cell cycling and reduced transplantation ability [8]; likewise, the inhibition of TGF-β in normal HSC with neutralizing antibodies releases cells into the cell cycle [9]. Inhibiting SMAD 4 signaling, key to TGF-β signaling, decreased HSC self-renewal in vivo [10]. The rapid generation of donor neutrophils that are the last cells to regenerate in bone marrow transplantation (BMT) is observed in transplanted mice after LTR-HSCs were treated with an antisense TGF-β1 PMO [6].

Phosphorodiamidate morpholino oligomers (PMOs) resist degradation [11], enhance specificity through a no-pucker six-membered morpholine ring in place of the five-membered ribose or deoxyribose [12], and are net charge neutral with one non-bridging oxygen substituted with a dimethylamine residue [13]. PMOs binds to the target RNA, forming a PMO:RNA heteroduplex that can inhibit translation [14] or pre-mRNA splicing [15]. The cellular internalization of PMOs in different cell types is mixed and not robust unless entry is assisted by cell uptake technologies [16]. Given the impressive safety profile for unmodified PMO [17–19], conjugation with delivery enhancements adds risk. An unmodified PMO represents the most specific and least risk to the modulation of gene expression in HSC.

Antisense TGF-β will reverse HSC growth arrest induced by TGF-β ligand, informing the reversibility of the ligand [20]. The antisense approach gains access to autocrine RNA expression over neutralizing antibodies, which targets protein. Transient antisense inhibition of autocrine TGF-β1 in HSC triggers a cascade of hematopoietic proliferation and differentiation that paracrine TGF-β cannot alter [21]. We report the kinetics of HSC internalization and efflux of PMO essential to transient inhibition of TGF-β1.

2. Feasibility: PMO entry into CD34+ stem cells

Evidence for receptor-mediated internalization of DNA came from studies with leukocytes over 30 years ago [22]. Uptake involves endocytosis based on chloroquine, a lysosomotropism agent, enhanced intracellular fluorescence, sodium azide inhibited internalization, and a punctate pattern observed in the cytoplasm [23]. Scavenger receptors on rat liver endothelial cells participate in uptake and play a prominent role in plasma clearance [24]. Many oligonucleotide uptake pathways have been described, but the adaptor protein AP2 M1 is involved in phosphorothioate oligonucleotide (PSO) uptake. siRNA targeting clathrin and caveolin had no effect on antisense activity but did decrease the uptake of fluorescently labeled oligonucleotides, highlighting multiple subcellular compartments that accumulate oligonucleotides but not all are associated with antisense activity. Abasic oligomers, backbone and sugar without nucleobase oligomers, were not transported into cells by the AP2 M1 pathway [25], pointing to the nucleobase as a recognition site for uptake. The neutral charge of PMO compounds sets them apart from ionic forms like PSO.

We explored techniques to deliver PMO into cells in culture to improve bioavailability and efficacy including scrape loading [26], syringe loading [27], microinjection [28], osmotic loading [29], and complexation with cationic lipids [30]. These techniques suffer from limited efficiency and poor reproducibility and often leave residual biologically active carrier molecules in the culture media. We then explored a variety of cationic peptides conjugated to the PMO for an enhanced delivery including HIV-TAT [31] and a broad spectrum of arginine-rich peptides [32–34]. At present, the optimal delivery peptide is still composed of multiple arginines [35]. A concern for loading arginine into a stem cell was the role arginine plays in generating NO, a complication in interpreting observations of CD34+ activation. Thus, we examined unassisted entry in stem cells.

Earlier studies evaluating unassisted PMO entry into cultured cells revealed that primary cell cultures are more efficient in uptake than established cell lines. Uptake is independent of PMO sequence or the position of FITC conjugation (5′ vs. 3′ ends are equivalent) (**Figure 1A**) but dependent on concentration (**Figure 1B**), time, and temperature. There is a direct relationship between fluorescence intensity of CD34+ cells and PMO concentration. Localization to both cytoplasmic and nuclear compartments is observed, so that both pre-mRNA and mRNA targets are feasible. Uptake into hematopoietic lineages reveals that monocytes and dendritic cell uptake are efficient, while entry into CD8+ T-cells, CD4+ T-cells, and B-cells is minimal [36]. Viral infection activates some T-cell populations, resulting in permissive PMO uptake [37]. Current understanding of mechanisms involved in activation associated with PMO uptake is limited.

The first evidence of unassisted PMO entry into CD34+ cells came from microscopic observation of cells in which the visible uptake of FITC-PMO came within 15 min. Stem cells are unique in permissive unassisted PMO uptake. The maximal saturation of PMO uptake into HSC occurs within 2 h (**Figure 2**). Optimal uptake in terms of activation of HSC occurs after 16 h of FITC-PMO incubation. Stem cell positivity after 16 h was observed at 37°C with 70 ± 12% FITC-positive CD34+ cells (n = 6), room temperature incubation led to 56 ± 8% positive cells (n = 5), and 4°C incubation led to 30 ± 19% positive cells (n = 6). The percent FITC-PMO-positive CD34+ cells were mirrored by cellular fluorescence defined by mean channel fluorescence with 112 ± 47 at 37°C, 56 ± 22 at room temperature, and 31 ± 24 at 4°C incubation. Negative controls included CD34+ cells incubated with no FITC-PMO at 4°C, RT, and 37°C (n = 6) for each group, and no FITC-PMO-positive cells were observed.

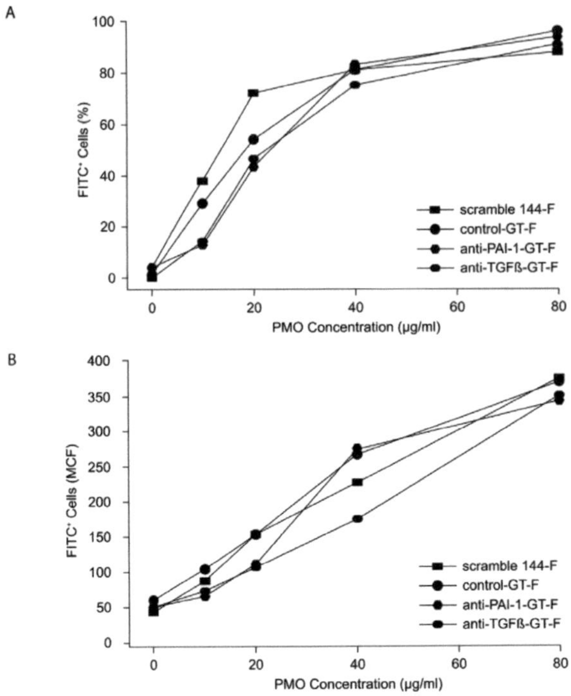

Figure 1. Concentration-dependent uptake of FITC-PMO into CD34+ human stem cells. A. Percent-positive CD34+ HSC on the ordinate and PMO concentration on the abscissa. B. Mean channel fluorescence of CD34+ HSC on the ordinate and PMO concentration on the abscissa. The uptake of PMOs is not sequence specific: 20-mer PMOs have similar entry kinetics, and percent-positive CD34+ cells are directly proportional to the PMO concentration in the medium. CD34+ cells were isolated from the blood of healthy subjects by pre-enriching the CD34+ by a lineage negative selection followed by FACS sorting of CD34+ CD45+ cells.

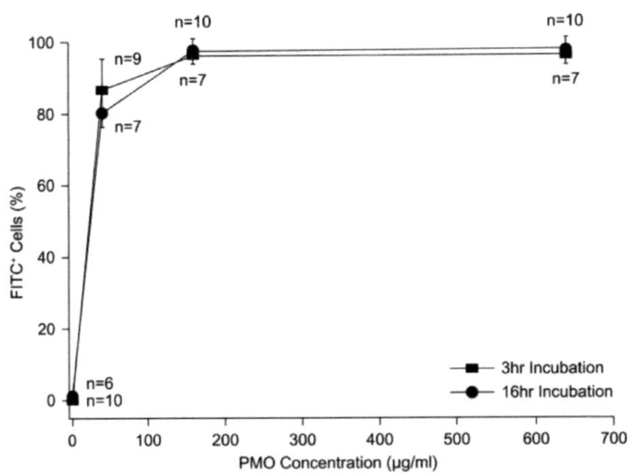

Figure 2. Time-dependent uptake of FITC-PMO into CD34+ human stem cells. After 3 h at 37°C at 150 µg/mL 144-F (a FITC-control PMO), >95% of CD34+ cells became FITC-labeled. At 16 h in culture, the degree of FITC-144-F PMO was the same as the 3-h point. CD34+ cells were isolated and FACS sorted from the blood of healthy subjects as described in **Figure 1**.

http://dx.doi.org/10.5772/intechopen.79650

PMO uptake was found to be time and dose dependent. Uptake reached 100% FITC-PMO-positive CD34+ cells between 1 and 6 h of incubation at 37°C. Uptake determined as percent-positive CD34+ cells measured over time were linear (r2 0.94–0.94) (**Table 1**). Comparison of CD34+ cells recovered from diabetic individuals to non-diabetic individuals reveals that uptake is three to five times more rapid in non-diabetic CD34+ cells compared to those from diabetic individuals (**Table 1**, **Figure 3**). No loss in cell viability has been observed in protocols involving a 6-h incubation sufficient for 100% PMO-positive cells. Preliminary data suggest that treated stem cells will carry less than 5 μg PMO into the eye as a result of a combination of

Treatment group	Rate percent pos./H (r^2)[c]	Ratios (expected)	Time to 100% pos.	Saturation ratio
Norm[a] 40 μg (N = 2)	17.6 ± 1.1 (0.95)	3.3 (N/D 40)	6 h	3.0 (D/N 40)
Diab[b] 40 μg (N = 1)	5.3 ± 5.2 (0.95)	3.4 (D 160/40) [4]	18 h	3.6 (D 40/160) [4]
Norm 160 μg (N = 2)	98.0 ± 7.3 (0.94)	5.6 (N 160/40) [4]	1 h	6.0 (N 40/160) [4]
Diab 160 μg (N = 1)	18.1 ± 8.2 (0.94)	5.4 (N/D 160)	5 h	5.0 (D/N 160)

[a]CD34+ cells recovered from normal donors.
[b]CD34+ cells recovered from diabetic donors.
[c]Correlation coefficient from linear regression analysis.

Table 1. PMO uptake kinetics in CD34+ cells.

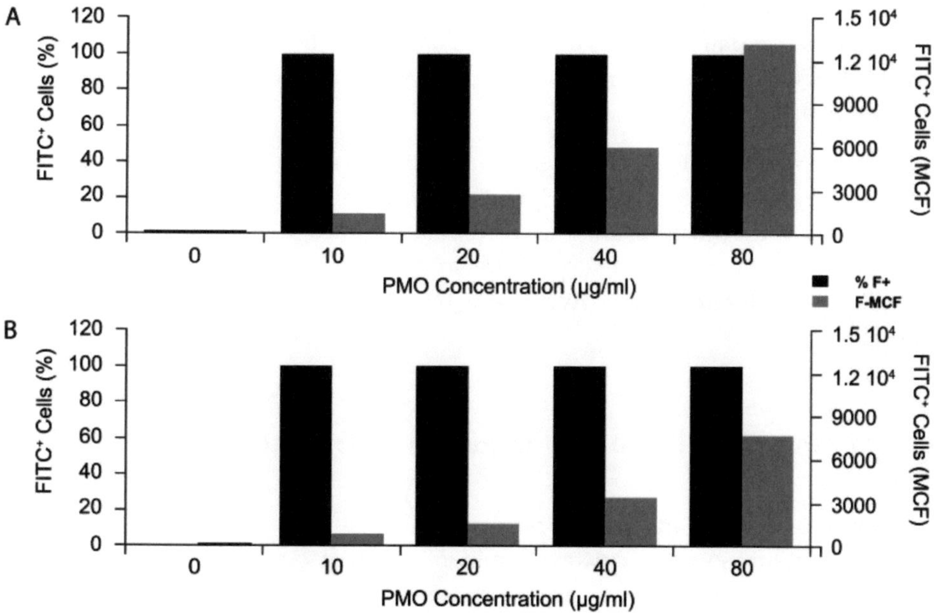

Figure 3. The percent of blood-derived CD34+ cell taking up FITC-PMO. A. Percent-positive (black bar) and mean channel fluorescence (gray bar) CD34+ cells from healthy donors. B. Percent-positive (black bar) and mean channel fluorescence (gray bar) CD34+ cells from diabetic subjects. Uptake is not different in healthy and diabetic subjects, but the rates of maximum saturation of FITC-PMO (measure by MEAN CHANNEL FLUORECENCE) are delayed in diabetic CD34+ cells relative to non-diabetic cells. CD34+ cells were pre-enriched and FACS sorted as described above.

efflux out of the cell, and tissue half-life will quickly lead to undetectable PMO and a transient inhibition of TGF-β in the stem cells. The overall exposure of PMO will be below 100,000 times the reported no observed adverse effect level (NOAEL) for a similar PMO in GLP toxicology studies [38, 39]. The use of PMO-treated CD34+ stem cells to treat patients with diabetic retinopathy is expected to be safe and feasible.

3. Optimal TGF-β PMO inhibitors in human Lin-CD34+ CD45+ HSC

TGF-β is a family of multifunctional peptide cytokines with the capacity to regulate proliferation, differentiation, adhesion, migration, and other functions in many cell types. TGF-β receptors are found on most cells, and their signal transduction positively and negatively regulates many other growth factors. Secreted TGF-β is cleaved into a latency-associated peptide (LAP) and a mature TGF-β1 protein. TGF-β is latent in the form of a TGF-β1 homodimer, a LAP homodimer, and a latent TGF-β1-binding protein (LTBP). However, TGF-β1 homodimer can be active, and the mature protein may also form heterodimers with other TGF-β family members.

The HSC is pluripotent immature cell that can generate daughter cells committed to all nine types of mature blood cells, including trillions of white blood cells, red blood cells, and platelets. HSCs are found in the bone marrow and also circulate in the peripheral blood. HSC possesses two key properties: (1) the ability to self-renew (generating HSC replicates) and (2) the ability to generate daughter cells that differentiate into fully functional blood cells (namely, asymmetrical HSC division in which one daughter cell remains a HSC and the other daughter cells are destined to mature).

When the most primitive HSCs self-replicate, they produce daughter cells with a long (possibly unlimited) clonal life span. When HSC replication leads to differentiation divisions, they lose their multi-lineage potential and the corresponding lineage commitment accompanied by a progressive reduction in clonal life span. Previous studies have shown that *ex vivo* proliferation of HSC favors differentiation divisions at the expense of self-replication, resulting in a complete loss of HSC.

4. TGF-β is an optimal stem cell target for CD34+ stem cells

An inhibitor of c-myc was identified based on antiproliferative effects in differentiated cells that block translation as well as create a dominant-negative variant of c-myc [40]. This inhibitor was effective in preventing coronary restenosis [41], preventing cyst growth in kidneys of polycystic kidney disease models [42], and reducing tumor growth [43]. We investigated the c-myc inhibitor in c-kit+/sca-1+ cells incubated with IL-3, IL-6, and SCF to drive cell proliferation of the stem cells. Incubation of these cells with saline was associated with a cell doubling half-life of 2.66 days, a scrambled sequence PMO (5′-GCTATTACCTTAACCCAG-3′) had a doubling half-life of 2.554 days, and the c-myc inhibitor (5′-ACGTTGAGGGGCATCGTCGC-3′)

had a doubling half-life of 2.53 days. Unlike differentiated cells, the stem cells show no difference in cell proliferation when c-myc was inhibited. While inhibiting, *c-myc* did not influence proliferation rate; however, it did enhance stem cell differentiation as high proliferation potential (HPP) colony forming counts (CFC) rose from 3.8 HPP CFC in controls to 8.0 HPP-CFC in *c-myc*-inhibited cultures. This surprising observation suggested that *c-myc* inhibition stimulates stem cell differentiation and regulates self-renewal inspired studies to look at upstream signaling pathways in these stem cells. We studied the inhibition of ecotropic virus insertion-1 (EVI-1), which inserts in the DNA of murine stem cells and c-Kit, a stem cell marker along with c-myc and found that PMO-antisense treatment in vitro decreased LTR-HSC repopulating ability (**Figure 4**). Furthermore, the intra-peritoneal administration of PMO anti-c-myc reduces HSC-repopulating ability in vivo (**Figure 5**). These results represent an excellent functional control for PMO-TGF-β1 since these PMO antisense treatments do not promote HSC engraftment while PMO-TGF-β1 does.

ID11, a neutralizing monoclonal antibody to three isoforms of TGF- β (TGF- β1, 2, 3), added to stem cell cultures can replace growth factors and prevent apoptosis in mouse HSC [7]. Adding 100 c-kit+/sca-1+ cells to 96-well plates with no IL-3, IL-6, or SCF led to no cells observed after 5 days in culture. Adding ID11 to those cultures led to 37 ± 7 cells, confirming that the antibody could replace growth factors. Further, the addition of the PMO targeting *c-myc* led to 10 ± 3 cells at 5 days in culture, leading us to conclude that *c-myc* expression is required for the loss of TGF-β phenotype. It became apparent that ID11 effectively blocks extracellular TGF-β, but a PMO (5′-GCA CTG CCG AGA GCG CGA ACA-3′) inhibitor of TGF-β translation could have the advantage of blocking autocrine signaling. Inhibiting TGF-β with either antibody or antisense PMO enhances HPP-CFC from progenitor cells [7, 20, 21] and can enhance hematopoietic reconstitution following bone marrow transplantation [6, 44, 45]. Importantly,

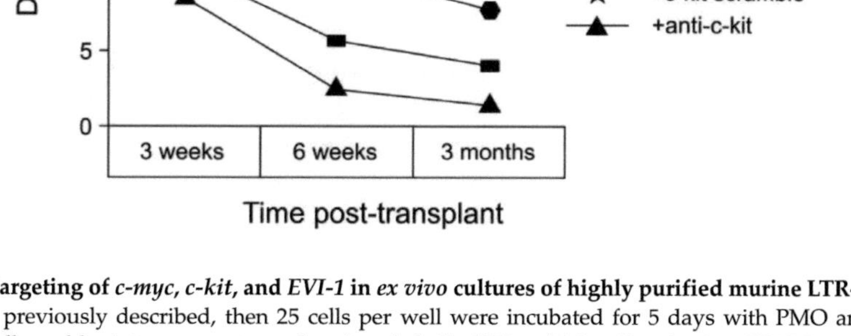

Figure 4. PMO targeting of *c-myc, c-kit,* and *EVI-1* in *ex vivo* cultures of highly purified murine LTR-HSC. LTR-HSCs were isolated as previously described, then 25 cells per well were incubated for 5 days with PMO and hematopoietic growth factors followed by intravenous transplant into lethally (950 rads) irradiated mice. CD45.2 congenic LTR-HSCs were transplanted into CD45.1 recipients, so that donor LTR-HSC could be detected by monoclonal antibodies. Significantly fewer ($p < 0.05$) LTR-HSCs were observed in cultures treated with *c-kit, EVI-1,* and *c-myc* PMO compared to control, c-myc scramble, and c-kit scramble PMO after 3 months post-transplant.

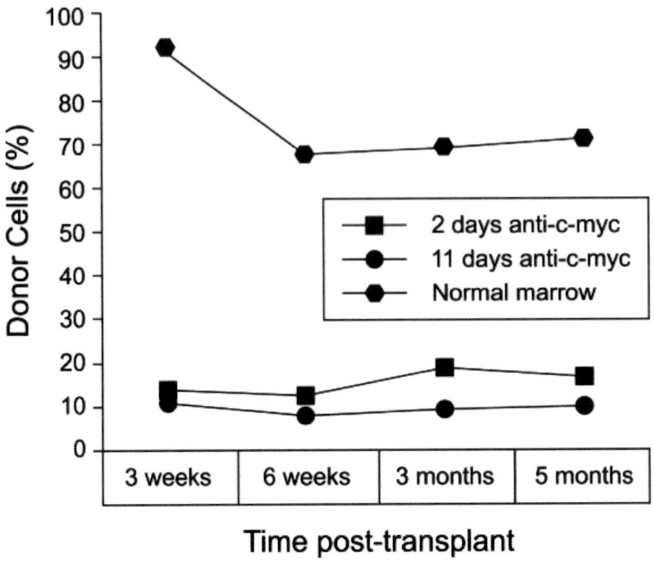

Figure 5. In vivo activity of PMO targeting *c-myc* in short-term and long-term hematopoietic stem cells. Mice were treated with *c-myc*-PMO in vivo (intraperitoneal injection) for 2 or 11 days. At each time point, mice were sacrificed, and the femoral marrow was assayed for HSC levels using a murine transplantation model. Significant reductions in repopulating HSC ($p < 0.05$) were observed in mice treated with c-myc PMO compared to normal bone marrow.

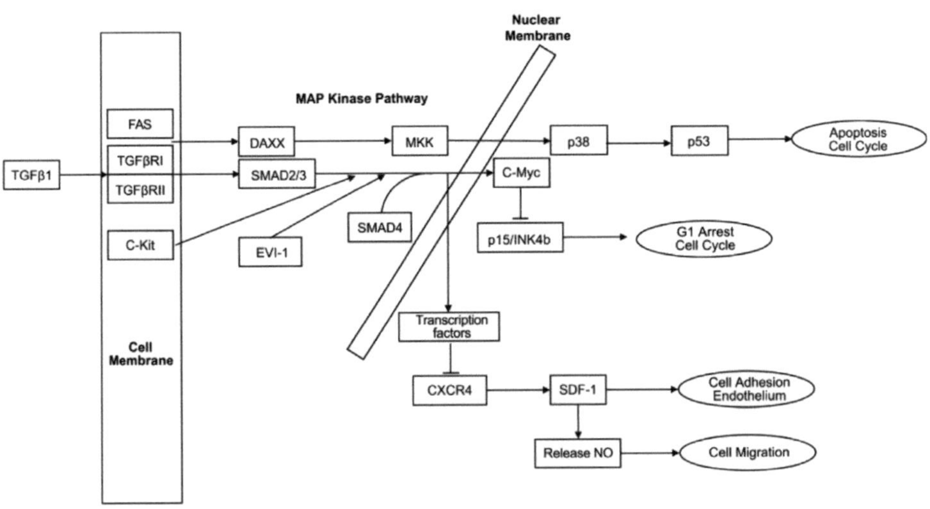

Figure 6. Targeting stem cell pathways. Studies were conducted targeting c-myc, SMAD4, EVI-1, c-kit, TGF-βRI, TGF-βRII, and TGF-β1 with PMOs designed to inhibit expression in HSC. Regulation of transcription factors by TGF-β1 is linked to stem cell homing through CXCR4 interaction with SDF-1 and release of nitric oxide and elevated migration. The MAP kinase pathway signaling reveals the potential mechanism for the prevention of apoptosis with TGF-β1 inhibition. The upstream regulation of c-myc and p53 by TGF-β1 inhibition allows stem cells to proliferate. Inhibition of TGF-β1 is the optimal target resulting in stem cell proliferation, homing, and migration of all favorable properties for autologous transplantation.

the transplantation of Tfgβ1$^{-/-}$ bone marrow into lethally radiated TGF-β1$^{+/+}$ recipients reconstitutes all hematopoietic lineages [46]. Taken together, these studies encouraged further examination of the TGF-β1-signaling pathway.

We investigated PMO inhibitors of TGF-β receptor I (5′CAT GGT CCC TGC AGA GAG GA-3′) and TGF-β receptor II (5′-GAC CCA TGG CAG CCC CCG TCG-3′) to reveal the same phenotype to the TGF-β1 ligand inhibitor. Subsequent studies targeting SMAD 4 (5′-AAT CAT ACT CAT CCT TCA CCA TCA T-3′) also led to the TGF-β-inhibited phenotype in CD34+ cells, confirming that the signal transduction pathway is responsible for the phenotype, while blocking other pathways did not (**Figure 6**). We focused on the TGF-β1 ligand due to the short half-life, enabling rapid onset and transient inhibition properties of the treatment.

5. The optimal TGF-β1 inhibitor

We investigated the use of an antisense PMO targeting the AUG translation start site for efficacy in inhibiting TGF-β1 expression by hybrid arrest of translation. One possible outcome of a PMO at AUG1 will be for translation slippage to a translation initiation start site at amino acid 38, AUG38 (**Figure 7**). The resulting protein will not have the signal peptide, leading to the loss of appropriate subcellular localization, altered autocrine regulation, and possibly a protein with a shorter half-life. The diminished protein product fails to provide a negative feedback to the promoter, so enhanced transcription is expected. To test this hypothesis, we evaluated six oligomers targeting translation and two scrambled control sequences (**Table 2**).

The compounds were evaluated in an in vitro translation assay using rabbit reticulocyte lysate and a luciferase fusion transcript with TGF-β1 mRNA. Each of the antisense PMOs effectively inhibited translation, and the scrambled control oligomers did not inhibit, confirming PMO sequence specificity. The TGF-β1 PMO included 13 guanines (G) in the 20-mer and presented water solubility limitations and reduced synthetic yield concerns. Replacing guanine with inosine improved both water solubility and synthetic yield. However, inosine pairing with cytosine involves two hydrogen bonds in contrast to the three hydrogen bonds between guanine and cytosine. The hypothesis is that the more inosine replacement of guanine in the oligomer will result in a lower binding energy between PMO and target RNA and subsequent

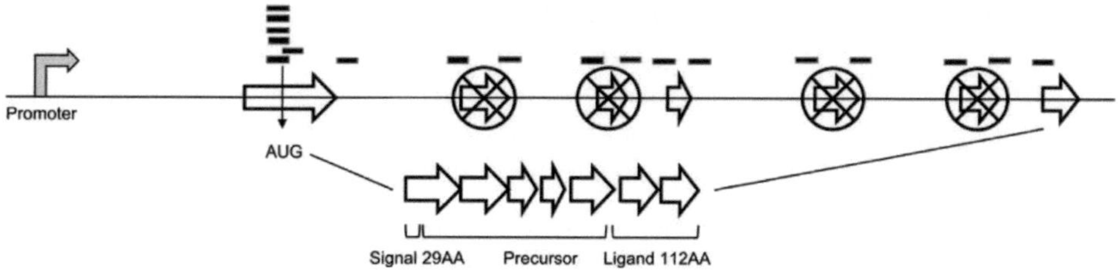

Figure 7. Optimal antisense strategy. Multiple PMOs were developed to inhibit translation initiation at the AUG site as well as targeting each exon at both splice donor and splice acceptor sites (black bars). Skipping exons 2, 3, 5, and 6 results in out-of-frame reading, and a nonsense-mediated decay (NMD) of the transcript is expected (X circles).

Name	Sequence 5′ → 3′	Mol Wt.
GT Control	CCTCCTACCTCAGTTACAATTTATA	—
144 Control	AGTCTCGACTTGCTACCTCA	7020
TGF-β1 GT	GCACTGCCGAGAGCGCGAACA	7642
TGF-β1	GAGGGCGG**CAT**GGGGGAGGC	7175
TGF-β1 1-I*	GAGGGCGG**CAT**GG I GGAGGC	7160
TGF-β1 3-I (1067)	GAGGGCGG**CAT**G III GAGGC	7130
TGF-β1 2-I	GAG I GCGG**CAT**GG I GGAGGC	7145
TGF-β1 4-I	GAG I GCGG**CAT**G III GAGGC	7115

*I refers to inosine, a strategy to limit "purine clash."

Table 2. Oligomer sequences employed to inhibit TGF-β1 translation.

diminished inhibition of translation. By contrast, the PMO with three inosines, TGF-β1 3-I (1067), inhibited translation more effectively than PMOs with all guanine or PMOs in which one or two guanines were replaced by inosine (data not shown).

TGF-β1 has seven exons transcribed into eight variant mRNAs, five alternately spliced variants and three unspliced forms (**Figure 7**). A small signal peptide (29 amino acids) is encoded in exon 1; the precursor LAP is encoded in exons 1 through 5; the active TGF-β1 is encoded in exons 6 and 7. The LTBP is encoded by a separate gene and binds directly to the LAP in the latent TGF-β complex prior to secretion. The amino terminus of LTBP binds to the extracellular matrix followed by proteolytic cleavage by a serine protease, plasmin, releasing the latent complex. A urokinase plasminogen activator (uPA) protease cuts the 391-amino acid TGF-β1 propeptide liberating the active 112 amino acid TGF-β1, which forms a homodimer ligand for the TGF-β receptors [47].

The TGF-β N terminal domain is present in a variety of proteins, which include TGF-β, decapentaplegic peptides, and bone morphogenetic proteins. The N-terminal domain expressed on the decapentaplegic protein acts as an extracellular morphogen guiding: (1) the proper development of the embryonic dorsal hypoderm, (2) viability of larvae, and (3) cell viability of the epithelial cells in the imaginal disks. When the N terminal domain is expressed on the bone morphogenetic protein (BMP), it induces cartilage and bone formation, possibly for epithelial osteogenesis. TGF-β1 is a protein composed of 112 amino acid residues liberated by proteolytic cleavage from the C-terminal of a precursor protein. A number of proteins are related to TGF-β1. The TGF-beta family is only active as homo- or heterodimers, the two chains being linked by a disulphide bond. X-ray studies of TGF-β2 reveal that all the other cysteines are involved in intrachain disulphide bonds. The four disulphide bonds in TGF-β and in the inhibin beta chains distinguish function from the other members of this family that lack the first bond. Concern has been noted as TGF-β not only exerts tumor-suppressive effects but also modulates cell invasion and immune regulation such that dysregulation of the TGF-β signaling pathway can result in tumor development.

In order to demonstrate PMO inhibition, THP-1 cells, which are human monocytes that express TGF-β, were studied. THP-1 grows equally well in RPMI supplemented with 10% fetal bovine serum and serum-free media. When grown in serum-free media, TGF-β is not secreted into the media (ELISA = 0 pg./mL). Media supplemented with 50 ng/mL PMA lead to TGF-β secretion (ELISA = 92 pg./mL). The addition of 10 μM atorvastatin (Lipitor) enhances TGF-β secretion by fivefold (ELISA >500 pg./mL) following 72 h of incubation.

The evaluation of mRNA from splice altering PMOs is shown (**Table 3**). The control fragment appears at the correct size. Cells treated with PMOs targeting SD Ex2, SD Ex4, and AUG show no variation in transcript size and thus no evidence of exon skipping. The AUG signal appears to be enhanced relative to the untreated control, possibly indicating a rebound induction of transcription. This may be anticipated as the translation start site inhibitor will lead to suppression of the propeptide including LAP, which may lead to loss of the negative feedback mechanism for TGF-β1 transcription. Cells treated with PMOs targeting SD Ex5 and SD Ex6 reveal smaller transcripts in addition to faint bands at the correct size. The SD Ex5 smaller transcript is consistent in size with the loss of exon 4 (74 bp), which would leave the mature mRNA in frame. Those transcripts skipping exon 5 would be smaller yet (148 bp) and are expected to be degraded by a nonsense-mediated decay (NMD), so that the product would not be observed. The SD Ex6 smaller fragment is approximately 800 bp in size, which is 300 bp smaller than the expected full-length transcript and consistent with loss of both exons 5 (148 bp) and 6 (156 bp), which would be 304 bp smaller than the full-length transcript.

Treatment (5 μM 96 h)	**Hu TGF-β1 protein (pg/mL)**	**Mu TGF-β1 protein (pg/mL) 5 μM 65 h**	**Cell viability (% control)**
No PMO	520 ± 2	—	100
Scr Ctr	502 ± 15	1700 ± 10	88
SD Ex1*	385 ± 7	—	—
SA Ex2	387 ± 5	—	—
SD Ex2	BLD	1320 ± 30	93
SA Ex3	594 ± 21	—	—
SD Ex3	222 ± 3	—	—
SA Ex4	465 ± 12	—	—
SD Ex4	23 ± 2	520 ± 20	66
SA Ex5		—	—
SD Ex5	BLD	120 ± 10	79
SA Ex6	404 ± 18	—	—
SD Ex6	BLD	330 ± 10	79
SA Ex7	101 ± 1	—	91

*SD refers to the splice donor site of the exon (Ex) and SA refers to the splice acceptor site.

Table 3. Exon skipping in THP-1 cells stimulated to secrete TGF-β1.

Skipping exon 6 alone or exon 5 alone would be degraded by NMD, and those transcripts would not be observed. Skipping exons 5 and 6 will also remain in frame.

The exercise to identify an optimal inhibitor of TGF-β1 involved screening multiple gene targets and dozens of PMO inhibitors. Qualitative differences between splice-altering strategies and translation inhibitors involve the preservation of feedback inhibition of the promoter. Translation inhibitors and splice-altering targets that induce a nonsense-mediated decay (NMD) prevent the synthesis of the negative feedback, resulting in compensatory transcription followed by rebound translation of TGF-β1. By contrast, skipping of exons 5 and 6 leads to translation products with altered function but includes the LAP portion of the translated product, resulting in a prolonged inhibition of TGF-β1. Transient inhibition of TGF-β1 is desired [48], so the optimal approach favors the AUG and NMD PMO over exon skipping and ligand-neutralizing antibodies. Translation inhibition is preferred over NMD because NMD responses may be less reliable.

6. Stem cell therapy for diabetic retinopathy

The Centers for Disease Control and Prevention report that 4.2 million (28.5%) of US diabetics aged ≥40 years have diabetic retinopathy (DR) or damage to the small blood vessels in the retina that may result in loss of vision [49]. The direct costs for DR in the US were over $4.5 billion, and the indirect economic impact was an additional $5 billion. Retinopathy occurs in almost all patients with type 1 diabetes and 75% of patients with type 2 diabetes within 15 years of the manifestation of diabetes [50]. Over 12,000 diabetic patients become blind each year due to ocular complications [51]. Current therapy addresses the end stages of DR including laser photocoagulation, intravitreal antivascular endothelial growth factor (VEGF) agents such as Bevacizumab and Aflibercept, intravitreal corticosteroids such as Triamcinolone, and vitreoretinal surgery. CD34+ stem cells from diabetic patients cannot generate endothelial cells to repair the vasculature, instead generating more inflammatory monocytes [52]. The CD34+ stem cell therapy described here exploits the ability of these cells to differentiate into a wide variety of cell types to stimulate both vascular and neural regeneration to treat early stages of DR.

CD34+ cells are capable of homing to vascular lesions in the eye, mediating vascular repair [53]. The use of autologous CD34+ cells eliminates the significant complication of transplant rejection. However, diabetic CD34+ cells are dysfunctional, contributing to the diabetic complication of DR [54]. While CD34+ cells from healthy subjects could repair retinal capillaries in streptozotocin-induced diabetic mice, spontaneously diabetic obese BBZDR/Wor rats and neonatal mouse oxygen-induced retinopathy animal models CD34+ cells from diabetic mice could not [55]. The approach described here restores function to dysfunctional diabetic CD34+ cells.

TGF-β1 is overexpressed and may cause dysfunction in diabetic CD34+ cells, and correction of this overexpression can restore the regenerative ability of those cells in diabetics. TGF-β1 is the major regulator of the balance between CD34+ proliferation, differentiation, and quiescence. Transient inhibition of TGF-β1 with an optimal PMO (1) activates human CD34+ proliferation, whereas ID11 antibody does not, (2) enhances CXCR4 cell surface expression and effective stem cell homing to SDF-1 ligand, (3) increases nitric oxide (NO) release, stimulating stem cell migration, and (4) increases vascular repair by the activated diabetic CD34+ cells. The transient TGF-β1 inhibition approach holds potential to impact other diabetic microvascular complications and improve current bone marrow transplantation processes used in the treatment of blood cancers.

The transient inhibition of TGF-β1 in autologous diabetic CD34+ cells with an antisense PMO ex vivo represents a feasible approach that poses minimal potential for adverse events and has potential benefit to the patient with diabetic retinopathy. Challenges remain in development such as the selection of animal models that adequately predict the human response to treatment. Numerous features including the genetic basis of the retinal disease, anatomical differences in the eye, and the genesis of retinal damage limit the utility of animal models. Substantial differences in diabetic subpopulations, the presence of comorbidities, patient age, and diabetes severity will influence the success of our proposed therapy. A detailed understanding of the natural history of diabetic retinopathy deserves in-depth investigation, so that patient enrollment can be refined, and clinical trials will examine optimal patient populations and appropriate stage of disease. Current efforts are ongoing to address these limitations as our protocol advances to the clinic.

7. Conclusions

Damaged retinal vessels are repaired by HSC in individuals throughout their life. Diabetic HSC function is impaired, leading to the development of numerous clinically important conditions including diabetic retinopathy. Selective *ex vivo* manipulation of TGF-β1 in diabetic HSC represents a therapeutic approach to maintain, enhance, and restore vascular viability in the retina. The PMO offers transcript selective binding and transient interference with translation of TGF-β1. The PMO offers a feasible technology in which they enter HSC, can inhibit autocrine TGF-β1 signaling in HSC, and have an excellent safety profile. We presented the process of selecting TGF-β1 as an optimal transcript and the optimal PMO sequence targeting TGF-β1 mRNA. Our studies identified a transient interference with the translation of TGF-β1 in diabetic CD34+ HSC with an antisense PMO that will (1) upregulate the expression of CXCR4, enabling stem cell homing and adhesion to sites of vascular injury in the retina, (2) stimulation of nitric oxide production, enabling stem cell mobility, and (3) the release of cell cycle checkpoints, enabling stem cell proliferation and differentiation required for the repair of vascular lesions. The manipulated stem cell treatment strategy is making the transition from discovery to preparation for clinical evaluation.

Acknowledgements

We acknowledge the exacting experimentation performed by Dr. Ewa Sitnicka and Carl Storey for the murine stem cell/transplantation studies. We also thank Valerie Stepps and Casey Renée Haynes for their persistent, successful efforts, exploring the uptake of FITC-PMO by highly enriched CD34+ cells. Finally, the extensive effort made by Elizabeth Bartelmez to help prepare numerous NIH proposals is also gratefully acknowledged. These studies were primarily funded by NIH grants awarded to SB (NIH NIDDK, R01 DK48708; R43 HL093955 NIH/NHLB; R43 HL093955 EY; RC1 EY020341 NIH/NEI; 1R44EY028070-01).

Conflict of interest

The authors of this chapter have financial interest in BetaStem Therapeutics, Sausalito CA.

Author details

Patrick L. Iversen[1]*, Francis W. Ruscetti[2], Charles Garcia[3] and Stephen H. Bartelmez[4]

*Address all correspondence to: patmanphd@gmail.com

1 Oregon State University, University of Oregon, and LS Pharma, Grand Junction, Colorado, USA

2 M.A.R.C. Inc., Carlsbad, CA, USA

3 UT Medical School at Houston, Houston, TX, USA

4 BetaStem Therapeutics, Sausalito, CA, USA

References

[1] Becker A, McCullough E, Till J. Cytological demonstration of the clonal nature of spleen colonies derived from transplanted mouse marrow cells. Nature. 1963;**197**:452-454

[2] Robertson I, Hriguchi M, Zilberberg L, Dabovic B, Hadjiolova K, Rifkin D. Latent TGF-β-binding proteins. Matrix Biology. 2015;**47**:44-53

[3] Keller J, McNiece I, Sill K, Ellingsworth L, Quesenberry P, Sing G, Ruscetti F. Transforming growth factor-β directly regulates primitive murine hematopoietic cell proliferation. Blood. 1990;**75**:596-602

[4] Mamura M, Lee W, Sullivan T, Felici A, Sowers A, Allison J, Letterio J. CD28 disruption exacerbates inflammation in T-β1$^{-/-}$ mice: In vivo suppression of CD4+ CD25+ regulatory T cells independent of autocrine TGF-β1. Blood. 2004;**103**:4594-4601

[5] Mu Y, Gudey S, Landstrom M. Non-Smad signaling pathways. Cell and Tissue Research. 2012;**347**:11-20

[6] Bartelmez S, Storey C, Iversen P, Ruscetti F. Transient inhibition of endogenous transforming growth factor- β1 (TGFβ1) in hematopoietic stem cells accelerates engraftment and

enhances multi-lineage repopulating efficiency. Journal of Stem Cell Research and Therapy. 2016;**1**(7):00045

[7] Sitnicka E, Ruscetti FW, Bartelmez SH. Transforming growth factor-β1 (TGFβ1) directly and reversibly inhibits the initial cell division of long-term repopulating stem cells. Blood. 1996;**88**:82-88

[8] Yamazaki S, Ema H, Karlsson G, Yamaguchi T, Miyoshi H, et al. Nonmyelinating Schwann cells maintain hemtopoietic stem cell hibernation in bone marrow niche. Cell. 2011;**147**(5):1146-1158

[9] Imbert AM, Bagnis C, Galindo R, Chabannon C, Mannoni P. A neutralizing anti-TGF-beta-1 antibody promotes proliferation oc CD34+Thy-1+ peripheral blood progenitors and increases the number of transduced progenitors. Experimental Hematology. 1998;**26**(5):374-381

[10] Karlsson G, Blank U, Moody JL, Ehringer M, Singbrant S, Deng CX, Karlsson S. Smad4 is critical for self-renewal of hematopoietic stem cells. The Journal of Experimental Medicine. 2007;**204**(3):467-474

[11] Hudziak RM, Barofsky E, Barofsky DF, Weller DL, Huang SB, Weller DD. Resistance of morpholino phosphorodiamidate oligomers to enzymatic degradation. Antisense and Nucleic Acid Drug Development. 1996;**6**:267-272

[12] Stein D, Foster E, Huang SB, Weller DD, Summerton J. A specificity comparison of four antisense types: Morpholino, 2′-O-methyl RNA, DNA, and phosphorothioate DNA. Antisense and Nucleic Acid Drug Development. 1997;**7**:151-157

[13] Summerton J, Review Article WDD. Morpholino antisense oligomers: Design, Prepatation, and properties. Antisense and Nucleic Acid Drug Development. 1997;**7**:187-195

[14] Ghosh C, Stein D, Dwight Weller D, Iversen P. Methods for evaluation of antisense mechanisms of action. In: Phillips I, editor. Antisense Technology Part A, General Methods, Methods of Delivery, and RNA Studies. Methods in Enzymology. Vol. 313. San Diego, CA: Academic Press; 1999. pp. 135-142

[15] Giles RV, Spiller DG, Clark RE, Tidd DM. Antisense morpholino oligonucleotide analog induces missplicing of c-myc mRNA. Antisense and Nucleic Acid Drug Development. 1999;**9**:213-220

[16] Ghosh C, Iversen PL. Intracellular delivery stategies for antisense phosphorodiamidate morpholino oligomers. Antisense & Nucleic Acid Drug Development. 2000;**10**(4):263-274

[17] Sazani P, Weller DL, Shrewsbury SB. Safety pharmacology and genotoxicity evaluation of AVI-4658. International Journal of Toxicology. 2010;**29**(2):143-156. DOI: 10.1177/1091581809359206

[18] Sazani P, Van Ness KP, Weller DL, Poage DW, Palyada K, Shrewsbury SB. Repeat-dose toxicology evaluation in cynomolgus monkeys of AVI-4658, a phosphorodiamidate morpholino oligomer (PMO) drug for the treatment of duchenne muscular dystrophy. International Journal of Toxicology. 2011;**30**(3):313-321. DOI: 10.1177/1091581811403505

[19] Iversen PL, Newbry S. Manipulation of zebrafish embryogenesis by phosphorodiamidate morpholino oligomers indicates minimal non-specific teratogenesis. Current Opinion in Molecular Therapeutics. 2005;**7**(2):104-108

[20] Hatzfeld J, Li M, Brown E, Sookdeo H, Levesque J, O'Toole T, Gurney C, Clark S, Hatzfeld A. Release of early human hematopoietic progenitors from quiescence by antisense transforming growth factor β1 or Rb oligonucleotides. The Journal of Experimental Medicine. 1991;**174**:925-929

[21] Ruscetti FW, Akel S, Bartelmez SH. Autocrine transforming growth factor-β regulation of hematopoiesis: Many outcomes that depend on the context. Oncogene. 2005;**24**(37):5751-5763

[22] Bennett RM, Gabor GT, Merritt M. DNA binding to human leukocytes: Evidence for a receptor mediated association, internalization and degradation of DNA. The Journal of Clinical Investigation. 1985;**76**:2182-2190

[23] Loke SL, Stein CA, Zhang XH, Mori K, Nakanishi M, Subasinghe C, Cohen JS, Neckers LM. Characterization of oligonucleotide transport into living cells. Proceedings of the National Academy of Sciences of the United States of America. 1989;**86**:3474-3478

[24] Bijsterbosch MK, Manoharan M, Rump ET, DeVrueh RLA, van Veghel R, Tivel KL, Biessen EAL, Bennett CF, Cook PD, vanBerkel TJC. In vivo fate of phosphorothioate antisense oligodeoxynucleotides: Predominant uptake by scavenger receptors on endothelial liver cells. Nucleic Acids Research. 1997;**25**(16):3290-3296

[25] Koller E, Vincent TM, Chappell A, De S, Anoharan M, Bennett CF. Mehanisms of single-stranded phosphorothioate modified antisense oligonucleotide accumulation in hepatocytes. Nucleic Acids Research. 2011;**39**(11):4795-4807

[26] Partridge M, Vincent A, Matthews P, Puma J, Stein D, Summerton J. A simple method for delivering morpholino antisense oligos into the cytoplasm of cells. Antisense and Nucleic Acid Drug Development. 1996;**6**:169-175

[27] Ghosh C, Iversen PL. Intracellular delivery strategies for antisense phosphorodiamidate morpholino oligomers. Antisense and Nucleic Acid Drug Development. 2000;**10**:263-274

[28] Nasevicius A, Ekker SC. Effective targeted gene "knockdown" in zebrafish. Nature Genetics. 2000;**26**:216-220

[29] Wu-Pong S. Calcium-dependent oligonucleotide cellular uptake. Biochimie. 1996;**78**:33-38

[30] Morcos PA. Achieving efficient delivery of mopholino oligos in cultured cells. Genesis. 2001;**30**:94-102

[31] Moulton HM, Hase HC, Smith KH, Iversen PL. HIV Tat peptide enhances cellular delivery of antisense morpholino oligomers. Antisense & Nucleic Acid Drug Development. 2003; **13**:32-37

[32] Moulton HM, Nelson MH, Hatlevig SA, Reddy MT, Iversen PL. Cellular uptake of antisense morpholino oligomers conjugated to arginine-rich peptides. Bioconjugate Chemistry. 2004;**15**(2):290-299

[33] Abes S, Moulton HM, Clair P, Prevot P, Youngblood DS, Wu RP, Iversen PL, Lebleu B. Vectorization of morpholino oligomers by the (R-Ahx-R)(4) peptide allows efficient splicing correction in the absence of endosomolytic agents. Journal of Controlled Release. 2006; **116**(3):304-345

[34] Abes R, Arzumanov AA, Moulton HM, Abes S, Ivanova GD, Iversen PL, Gait MJ, Lebleu B. Cell-penetrating-peptide-based delivery of oligonucleotides: An overview. Biochemical Society Transactions. 2007;**35**(pt 4):775-779

[35] Echigoya Y, Nakamura A, Natata T, Urawawa N, Lim KRQ, Trieu N, Panesar D, Kuraoka M, Moulton HM, Saito T, Aoki Y, Iversen P, Sazani P, Kole R, Maruyama R, Partridge T, Takeda S, Yokota T. Effects of systemic multiexon skipping with peptide conjugated morpholinos in the heart of a dog model of duchenne muscular dystrophy. Proceedings of the National Academy of Sciences of the United States of America. 2017;**114**(16):4213-4218

[36] Iversen PL, Aird KM, Wu R, Morse MM, Devi GR. Cellular uptake of neutral phosphorodiamidate morpholino oligomers. Current Pharmaceutical Biotechnology. 2009;**10**(6): 579-588

[37] Schnell FJ, Sundholm S, Crumley S, Iversen PL, ad Mourich DV. Lymphocytic choriomeningitis virus infection in FVB mouse produces hemorrhagic disease. PLoS Pathogens. 2012;**8**(12):e1003073

[38] Sazani P, Ness KP, Weller DL, Poage D, Nelson K, Shrewsbury AS. Chemical and mechanistic toxicology evaluation of exon skipping phosphorodiamidate morpholino oligomers in mdx mice. International Journal of Toxicology. 2011;**30**(3):322-333

[39] Sazani P, Ness KP, Weller DL, Poage DW, Palyada K, Shrewsbury SB. Repeat-dose toxicology evaluation in cynomolgus monkeys of AVI-4658- a phosphorodiamidate morpholino oligomer (PMO) drug for the treatment of duchenne muscular dystrophy. International Journal of Toxicology. 2011;**30**(3):313-321

[40] Hudziak RM, Summerton J, Weller, Iversen PL. Antiproliferative effects of steric blocking phosphorodiamidate morpholino antisense agents directed against c-myc. Antisense & Nucleic Acid Drug Development. 2000;**10**:163-176

[41] Kipshidze N, Iversen P, Keane E, Stein D, Chawla P, Skrinska V, Shankar LR, Mehran R, Chekanov V, Dangas G, Komorowski R, Haudenschild C, Khanna A, Leon M, Keelan MH, Moses J. Complete vascular healing and sustained suppression of neointimal thickening after local delivery of advanced c-myc antisense at six months follow-up in a rabbit balloon injury model. Cardiovascular Radiation Medicine. 2002;**3**:26-30

[42] Ricker JL, Mata JE, Iversen PL, Gattone VH. C-myc antisense oligonucleotide treatment ameliorates murine infantile polycystic kidney disease. Kidney International. 2002;**61**: S125-S131

[43] Knapp DC, Mata JE, Reddy MT, Devi GR, Iversen PL. Resistance to chemotherapeutic drugs overcome by c-Myc inhibition in Lewis lung carcinoma model. Anti-Cancer Drugs. 2003;**14**(1):39-47

[44] Cardoso A, Li M, Batard P, Hatzfeld A, Brown E, Levesque J-P, Sookdeo E, Panterne B, Sansilvestri P, Clark S, Hatzfeld J. Release from quiescence of CD34+ CD38 human umbilical cord blood cells reveals their potentiality to engraft adults. Proceedings of the National Academy of Sciences of the United States of America. 1993;**90**:8707-8711

[45] Brenet F, Kermani P, Spektor R, Raffi S, Sandura J. TGF-ß restores hematopoietic homeostatis after chemotherapy. The Journal of Experimental Medicine. 2013;**210**:623-639

[46] Mamura M, Lee W, Sullivan T, Felici A, Sowers A, Allison J, Letterio J. CD28 disruption exacerbates inflammation in TGF-β1$^{-/-}$ mice: In vivo suppression by CD4+ CD25+ regulatory T cells independent of autocrine TGF-β1. Blood. 2004;**103**:4594-4601

[47] Gleizes PE, Munger JS, Nunes I, Harpel JG, Mazzieri R, Noguera I, Rifkin DB. TGF-β latency: Biological significance and mechanisms of action. Stem Cells. 1997;**15**:190-197

[48] National Diabetes Statistics Report. Centers for Disease and Control Department of Health and Human Services; 2014: www.cdc.gov/diabetes/pubs/statsreort14/national-diabetes-report-web.pdf

[49] Paine SK, Basu A, Mondal LK, Sen A, Choudhuri S, Chowdhury I, Saha A, Bhadhuri G, Mukerjee A, Bhattacharya B. Association of vascular endothelial growth factor, transforming growth factor beta, and interferon gamma gene polymorphisms with proliferative diabetic retinopathy in patients with type 2 diabetes. Molecular Vision. 2012;**8**:2749-2757

[50] American Diabetes Association: www.diabetes.org/living-with-diabetes/complications/eye-complications

[51] Otani A, Dorrell M, Kinder K, Moreno S, Nusinowitz S, Banin E, Heckenlively J, Friedlander M. Rescue of retinal degeneration by intravitreally injected adult bone marrow- derived lineage-negative hematopoietic stem cells. The Journal of Clinical Investigation. 2004;**114**:765-774

[52] Hazra S, Jarajapu Y, Steeps V, Caballero S, Thinschmidt J, Sautina L, Bengtsson N, Licalzi S, Dominguez J, Kern T, Segal M, Ash J, Saban D, Bartelmez SH, Grant MB. Long-term type 1 diabetes influnences hematopoietic stem cells by reducing vascular repair potential and increasing inflammatory monocyte generation in a murine model. Diabetologia. 2013; **56**(3):644-653

[53] Kijima H, Kim J, Chan L. Emerging roles of hematopoietic cells in the pathobiology of diabetic complications. Trends in Endocrinology and Metabolism. 2014;**25**:178-187

[54] Caballero S, Sengupta N, Afzal A, Chang KH, Li Calzi S, Guberski DL, Kern TS, Grant MB. Ischemic vascular damage can be repaired by healthy, but not diabetic, endothelial progenitor cells. Diabetes. 2007;**56**:960-967

[55] Bhatwadekar AD, Guerin E, Jarajapau Y, Caballero S, Sheridan C, Kent D, Kennedy L, Langsang MC, Ruscetti FW, Pepine C, Higgins P, Bartelmez SH, Grant MB. Transient inhibition of transforming growth factor-beta 1 in human diabetic CD34+ cells enhances vascular reparative functions. Diabetes. 2010;**59**:2010-2019

Section 2

Advances in Virotherapy: Virus-based Gene Therapy for Cancer and Other Genetic Diseases

Chapter 5

Gene-based Interventions for Cancer Immunotherapy

Otto L.D. Cerqueira,
Gissele Rolemberg Oliveira Silva,
Igor de Luna Vieira, Marlous Vinícius Gomes Lana,
Nadine Gimenez, Otavio Augusto Rodrigues,
Paulo Roberto Del Valle,
Samir Andrade Mendonça and Bryan E. Strauss

Additional information is available at the end of the chapter

http://dx.doi.org/10.5772/intechopen.80386

Abstract

Immunotherapy of cancer has deservedly gained much attention in the past few years and is likely to continue to advance and become a fundamental cancer treatment. While vaccines, chimeric antigen receptor (CAR) T cells and checkpoint blockade have received the lion's share of the attention, an important direct role for gene transfer as an immunotherapy is emerging. For example, oncolytic viruses induce immunogenic cell death, thus liberating both antigens and the signals that are necessary for the activation of antigen-presenting cells, ensuring stimulation of an adaptive response. In another example, transfer of prodrug converting enzymes, such as the herpes simplex virus-thymidine kinase (HSV-tk) gene or the cytosine deaminase gene, has been shown to promote an immune response, thus functioning as immunotherapies. Alternatively, our own work involves the use of nonreplicating viral vectors for the simultaneous delivery of gene combinations that promote both cell death and an immune response. In fact, our gene transfer approach has been applied as a vaccine, immunotherapy or *in situ* gene therapy, resulting in immunogenic cell death and the induction of a protective immune response. Here, we highlight the development of these approaches both in terms of technical advances and clinical experience.

Keywords: vaccine, CAR-T cell, oncolytic virotherapy, suicide gene, viral vectors

1. Introduction

The idea that the immune system acts as one of the barriers to the emergence and progression of tumors was conceived more than a 100 years ago [1]. Frank Macfarlane Burnet proposed the concept of "antitumor surveillance," which postulated that the immune system acted as a sentinel that controls and eliminates malignant cells [2]. This hypothesis was much debated and the lack of experimental evidence due to the technological limitations of the time generated a heated debate [3]. However, extensive data presented in the literature have since strengthened and expanded this concept [4–8].

The elaboration of appropriate immune responses must include the detection of the "self" and "nonself" antigens. For this, the immune system must not react to self-antigens and, at the same time, must detect threats to the organism, whether internal or exogenous. Tumors are particularly complex since these unwanted cells arise from the body's own tissues. Thus, upon detection of tumor cells, the immune system must strike a fine balance between activation of effector responses and tolerance. The immune system exploits the tenuous differences between normal cells in homeostasis and intrinsically related tumor cells.

Considering the high rate of mutation in tumors, the newly formed protein variants generate neoepitopes that may serve as targets for the detection and elimination of these aberrant and decontextualized cells by the immune system. These neoantigens can be, for example, the result of mutations caused by dysfunctional chromosomal recombination, such as the Philadelphia chromosome, generating a BCR-ABL gene fusion that did not previously exist in the body. This is a classic example of tumor-specific antigen (TSA), as seen in **Table 1**. Among the solid tumors, melanoma has the highest mutation rate (0.5 to >100 mutations per megabase), which reinforces the hypothesis that it is a highly immunogenic tumor [9]. Another characteristic of tumor cells is that they can express, or overexpress, genes outside the homeostatic context of their microenvironment, such tumor-associated antigens (TAAs) include oncofetal genes (linked to embryogenesis) or tissue markers, such as in melanoma (MAGE) or in breast cancer (HER2) [10]. These neoantigens and deregulated/overexpressed proteins are important targets for immunotherapeutic approaches.

Human tumor	**Antigenic protein**
Melanoma, esophageal and liver carcinoma	MAGE
Melanoma	Tyrosinase
Breast and ovarian carcinomas	HER2/Neu
Prostate carcinoma	Prostate-specific antigen (PSA)
Head-and-neck carcinoma	Caspase 8
Chronic myelogenous leukemia (CML)	BCR-ABL
Colon carcinoma	Carcinoembryonic antigen (CEA)

Table 1. Examples of TAA and TSA recognized by T cells.

Although antitumor immune responses do occur, tumors often develop elaborate strategies of evasion. This fundamental hallmark of cancer encompasses a wide variety of mechanisms and appears to exploit multiple levels and different cell types in the immune system, acting like a network. These mechanisms include (i) immunoediting, where the selection of variants of nonimmunogenic tumor cells (a phenomenon also known as immunoselection) is due to low expression of immunogenic molecules (like TAA) and/or major histocompatibility complex-I (MHC-I) molecules, and (ii) immuno-subversion, where immune suppressor signals are generated, thus disarming antitumor defenses [5, 7, 11].

These antitumor immune responses rely on innate and adaptive mechanisms. NK (natural killer) cells, part of the innate immune response, recognize MHC-I molecules (through the NKG2D receptor) and eliminate cells that have null or low expression. In addition, danger-associated molecular patterns (DAMPs) and stress-signaling proteins (MICA, MICB, ULBP4) signal an NK attack on cells that have suffered damage and that should be eliminated. Conditions such as irreparable levels of mutations and viral infections naturally trigger this signaling. However, the neoplastic cells can downregulate the expression of these stress markers and MHC-I or may secrete soluble MICA, thus avoiding NK cell attack [12].

Adaptive immunity also undergoes profound changes during tumor progression. Suppressive immune responses include the formation and recruitment of regulatory T lymphocytes (Treg), which, under normal conditions, inhibit the immune system's response to self-antigens [11]. In the tumor context, this mechanism is subverted to suppress antitumor immune responses, generating tolerance to tumor antigens [13–15]. These infiltrating Tregs contribute to the establishment of a tumor microenvironment abundant in immunosuppressive factors (IL-10, TGF-β, Arg1 and IDO) that influence many different cellular types, including the inhibition of effector T lymphocytes (Teff), generation of myeloid-derived suppressor cells (MDSC) and impairment of the proper function of dendritic cells (DCs) for presenting antigens [7].

The immunosuppressive tumor microenvironment also influences the immune checkpoint status, promoting the expression of inhibitory checkpoint molecules (CTLA-4, PD-1, IDO, LAG3, TIM3 and KIR) to the detriment of stimulatory checkpoint molecules (OX40, CD27, CD28, CD40, CD122 and ICOS) [16]. On the other hand, understanding this phenomenon brings interesting perspectives for immunotherapies as discussed below.

2. Immune interventions promoting active responses against tumor cells

Therapeutic strategies that target immune activation have shown significantly increased survival and quality of life for cancer patients [17]. Cancer immunotherapy comprises a variety of treatment approaches and combinations, incorporating the specificity of the adaptive immune response (T cells and antibodies) as well as the diverse and potent cytotoxic weaponry of both adaptive and innate immunity [18]. In this section, we provide an overview of key immunotherapeutic approaches.

Some of these strategies involve the application of soluble antibody molecules that specifically recognize and bind TAAs, resulting in blocked receptor signaling and/or passive immunotherapy. In particular, targeting tumor cells by engaging surface antigens differentially expressed in cancers has been widely used. For example, rituximab targets CD20 in non-Hodgkin B cell lymphoma. At least nine monoclonal antibodies (mAbs) targeting six TAAs (HER2/Neu, EGFR, VEGF, CD20, CD52 and CD33) are approved for the treatment of solid and hematological malignancies [19].

Approved by the Food and Drug Administration (FDA) in 2011, ipilimumab is a mAb against cytotoxic T lymphocyte–associated protein 4 (CTLA-4), a negative checkpoint of T cell function. Thus, checkpoint blockade with ipilimumab releases the brakes of the immune system, promoting T cells to combat cancer cells, and has already benefited thousands of patients with advanced melanoma, a disease that typically kills in less than a year [20]. Additional targets of immune checkpoint therapy include programmed cell death protein 1 (PD1) and its ligand PD-L1, which are even more effective and have fewer side effects as compared to anti-CTLA4 [21]. Moreover, checkpoint inhibitors may be used in combination with each other or with other therapies resulting in the induction of sustained antitumor responses in a wide variety of tumors [22–25]. Checkpoint blockade has undoubtedly been one of the most impressive advancements in cancer therapeutics in recent years, prolonging and saving the lives of many cancer patients. Even so, this approach does not directly induce a *de novo* immune response but releases experienced T cells from inhibitory signaling.

Vaccines are strategies to activate effector immune cells upon stimulation with tumor antigens, promoting the patient's own immune system to mount an immune response against neoplastic cells. Numerous vaccine approaches have been attempted and share the goal of providing effective target antigens while reverting, perhaps, the immunosuppressive tumor microenvironment and activating the ability of DCs to present these antigens. One example is GVAX (Cell Genesys, Inc., South San Francisco, CA), a polyvalent vaccine derived from a cultured cancer cell line expressing a plurality of shared tumor antigens. In addition, the cells have been genetically modified to secrete granulocyte-macrophage colony-stimulating factor (GM-CSF), an immune-modulatory cytokine that can activate antigen-presenting cells (APCs) locally at the vaccine site. Indeed, autologous and/or allogeneic GM-CSF-secreting tumor cell vaccines have demonstrated evidence of immunologic responses in patients with various types of cancers, for example, chronic myeloid leukemia [26], melanoma [27], pancreatic adenocarcinoma [28] and prostate cancer [29].

Oncolytic virotherapy (OV) is a novel form of cancer therapy that employs native or engineered viruses that selectively replicate in and kill cancer cells. OVs act as immunotherapies, promoting antitumor responses due to the viral infection of tumor cells and their acute lysis. An example of this therapy is an intralesional injection with talimogene laherparepvec (Imlygic, T-VEC, Amgen, Thousand Oaks, CA), a genetically engineered oncolytic HSV (herpes simplex virus), with mutations in infectious cell proteins (ICPs) 34.5 and 47, and expressing US11 and GM-CSF [30].

Alternatively, the patient's own T cells or NK cells may be used as a therapeutic agent. Such adoptive cell therapy (ACT) involves the recovery and *ex vivo* expansion of the patient's cells, providing the opportunity for selection and activation of tumor-specific populations, before they are infused in the patient [31]. One of the most advanced ACTs in clinical use is called CAR (chimeric antigen receptor) T cell therapy, which involves genetic modification of the patient's T cells to enhance their ability to recognize and attack cancer cells [32]. CAR-T cells have been engineered to express multiple CARs that recognize several tumor antigens. This technology has been successfully applied in clinical trials for hematological malignancies, with durable and complete remission in acute lymphoblastic leukemia [33], chronic lymphocytic leukemia [34] and B-cell lymphomas [35]. Another interesting application is the introduction of CARs targeting negative regulatory receptors, such as PD-1, resulting in reversal of immunosuppression in the tumor [36].

While cancer immunotherapies continue to evolve, the recurring role for gene transfer as a fundamental component of many of these approaches is quite evident. Here, we explore several immunotherapy approaches that rely on some aspects of gene transfer, highlighting both clinical and technological advances, especially as related to virotherapy, suicide genes, vaccines and CAR-T cells.

3. Cancer vaccines

Genetic instability intrinsic to cancer generates innumerable missense mutations in tumor cells and thus generates specific targets for T cell immunity [37]. Since these neoantigens are not expressed in normal somatic cells, they are inviting targets for the development of cancer vaccines and rational combinations of immunotherapies [38].

Although the term vaccine initially referred to the use of prophylactic immunizations for bacterial or viral infections, there are vaccines for therapeutic purposes, especially when we refer to cancer. This strategy has been gaining prominence lately as it offers the opportunity for a lasting effector response and with far fewer side effects than established traditional treatments, such as chemotherapy. In general terms, cancer vaccines seek to restore the ability of the immune system to recognize and eliminate neoplastic cells. In addition, the possibility of generating memory T cells favors long-lasting protective effects, including the prevention of metastasis after primary remission, which would greatly increase the survival and quality of life of these patients.

One of the earliest reports of cancer immunotherapy was conducted by William B. Coley. After observing that established tumors associated with fever or infection generally had higher rates of spontaneous regression, Streptococcus (Coley's toxin) was injected into an inoperable bone tumor. Despite generating data with difficult interpretation, it sparked a debate and numerous other fronts of investigation [39]. Corroborating this hypothesis, Lamm et al. demonstrated that Bacillus Calmette-Guerin (BCG) could be used to activate the immune system and thus enable the treatment of bladder cancer. This therapy, approved by the FDA, is still in clinical use [40].

3.1. Improving vaccine efficacy

In both of the pioneering works described above, bacterial components having immunostimulatory properties were used. It is now clear that the formulation of vaccines should include adjuvants, important components for immunomodulatory actions or acting as delivery systems for vaccine antigens [41–43]. The adjuvants' property of modulating the immune system is in part due to their interaction with the receptors of pathogen-associated molecular patterns (PAMPs). Toll-like receptor (TLR) and the Nod-like (nucleotide oligomerization domain) receptor families, for example, mediate the cellular response to PAMPs [44, 45]. Different classes of TLRs each recognize a specific molecular pattern. Briefly, TLRs 1, 2, 4, 5 and 6 recognize molecular patterns associated with bacteria. On the other hand, TLRs 3 and 7 are specialized in the recognition of molecular patterns associated with viral dsRNA and ssRNA, respectively. While TLRs 8, 9 and 13 recognize patterns of viruses and bacteria concomitantly, associated with ssRNA, DNA CpG patterns and ribosomal RNA sequences, respectively [46, 47]. The possibility of synergy when different innate receptors are stimulated may further enhance the adaptive immune response [48].

Several vaccine strategies may be employed for delivery of tumor antigens, adjuvants and modulators of the immune response (**Table 2**). Each strategy has its strengths and weaknesses. Even when meticulously planned, the actual response seen in clinical trials is often unpredictable. The vaccine regimen, number of doses, dosage, route of administration and adjuvant employed are variables that directly influence the type and intensity of the immune response generated. Another important point to be weighed is the mechanism of action, including (i) passive therapies based on the transfer of molecules (such as antibody or cytokine therapies) or mature immune effector cells for example transfer of adoptive T cells, or even CAR-T cell–based therapy; or, (ii) active therapies including classical therapeutic vaccines and those based on DCs to establish effector immune responses against tumors.

Protein-based immunotherapy combines peptides and/or proteins, aiming to activate antitumor immune responses. This strategy has been particularly effective in preventing oncogenic virus infection, as has been seen with Gardasil and Cervarix, which block HPV-associated cervical cancer [49]. The immune responses to structural proteins or viral oncoproteins are likely to be more effective since these antigens are foreign in the body. However, cancer-associated proteins or epitopes, being self-antigens, are naturally less immunogenic and typically associated with immune tolerance; consequently, they are less effective in eliciting immune responses in preclinical cancer models. In this way, delivery systems involving peptides, proteins and DNA/RNA vaccines, although classically used, may be poorly immunogenic and require appropriate pairing with adjuvants [50–52].

On the other hand, delivery systems based on viral vectors can be used for this purpose and may offer greater immunogenicity. Considering that many viral vectors come from pathogenic viruses such as lentivirus, retroviruses and adenoviruses, there is already a line of defense against these "intruders" that can be raised during immunotherapy. This strategy has inherent advantages, such as the possibility of activating innate immune responses due to a variety of viral molecular patterns that are agonists of TLRs, attracting and helping to mature cells of the adaptive immune response. As for the safety of these vectors, genetic engineering techniques allow the removal of specific genes related to pathogenicity, making them innocuous and safe for human use [53, 54]. In the last few years, several virus-driven therapies have been approved for human use, showing substantial progress in the field of gene therapy. Such approaches include Glybera for lipoprotein lipase deficiency and the oncolytic

Type	Generic mechanism	Clinical trials[a]	FDA approved
Protein based			
Peptides/proteins	Provide epitopes for specific antitumor immune responses.	446/278	Gardasil
Cytokine therapy	Modulate positively antitumor immunity.	721	Proleukin (IL2r)
Antibody therapy	Selectively target dysfunctional or overexpressed proteins in tumors.	4187	Rituximab, bevacizumab, ipilimumab, pembrolizumab
Gene based			
DNA/RNA vaccines	Provide epitopes for select antitumor immune responses.	142/80	–
Recombinant virus based			
Adenovirus	Gene transfer, including TK, CD and cytokines, among other transgenes.	193	–
Oncolytic virus	Selective infection in tumors promoting cell death.	74	Imlygic
Cell based			
Tumor cells	Provide wide range of epitopes for select antitumor immune responses.	78	–
Dendritic cells	Provide mature, activated and antigen-loaded dendritic cells for the correct antigen presentation, and consequent generation of effector T cells against the tumors.	574	Sipuleucel-T
Transfer of adoptive T cells	To provide T lymphocytes with lithic capacity directed at tumor cells.	77	–
CAR-T	T lymphocytes engineered *in vitro* that recognizes proteins/tumor epitopes, being endowed with lytic capacity independent of costimulatory molecules.	342	Kymriah

[a]clinicaltrials.gov, search performed April, 2018.

Table 2. Type of gene transfer used in vaccines and immunotherapy against cancer.

virotherapy Imlygic [55, 56], CAR-T cell immunotherapies Kymriah and Yescarta [57], as well as Strimvelis for the treatment of ADA-SCID (severe combined immunodeficiency due to adenosine deaminase deficiency) [58] and Luxturna for the treatment of Leber's congenital amaurosis [59].

The efficiency of immunotherapies may be increased by applying combinations of different strategies. The combination of antibody therapy, cytokine therapy and checkpoint blockade with other immunotherapeutic strategies has been shown to increase antitumor activity [60–62]. Antibody therapy often targets tumor antigens and/or tumor-promoting proteins. Some antibodies act as blockers of the function of their targets, while others may act as agonists. Additionally, the binding of these antibodies to their targets may direct opsonization or complement-mediated lysis and thereby contribute to the elimination of tumor cells. Another aspect of passive immune therapies is the use of recombinant cytokines, such as IL-2, IL-12 and interferon-α, β and γ [63]. Although both strategies can modulate the immune system to bring improvements, their action is temporary and can only be palliative, requiring successive doses and may provoke serious adverse effects [64, 65]. Checkpoint blockade has been gaining prominence recently and also encompasses the use of monoclonal antibody inhibitors of negative modulators of immune function, such as anti-PD-1, PDL1 and CTLA4 [66–68].

3.2. Modified dendritic cells as therapeutic vaccines

The presentation of antigens is a crucial event in the genesis of adaptive immune responses. Antigen-presenting cells (APCs) capture proteins in peripheral tissues, process them by proteolytic digestion and, after migrating to secondary lymphoid organs, present them to T lymphocytes in the context of class I or II MHC molecules [69]. In addition to the MHC molecules (HLA in humans), a number of costimulators (such as CD80, CD86, CD40, CD83 and CD14) are also required, important for the complementation of the biochemical signals necessary for the activation of T lymphocytes upon recognition of the presented antigens [70–72]. The maturation of cytotoxic T lymphocytes is central to the generation of adaptive immunity and, in turn, is one of the major antitumor defenses.

Autologous dendritic cell vaccines can be prepared from the patient's peripheral blood, with isolation of $CD14^+$ cells and *in vitro* treatment with GM-CSF and IL-4 for differentiation and maturation of monocyte-derived DCs (Mo-DCs). Next, different techniques can be used to "load" the tumor antigens into the DCs, such as peptides, proteins, DNA or RNA transfection, exosomes or exposure to tumor cell lysates [73, 74]. In addition to the changes that occur in the tumor microenvironment, the tumor is also capable of inducing systemic changes in the host's immune system, so that the monocytes from cancer patients may result in DCs with altered phenotype and cytokine production, negatively impacting immunotherapy [15]. Thus, immunotherapy with allogeneic DCs represents an interesting alternative. In addition to offering greater availability of DCs (since healthy donors have higher monocyte counts), tissue rejection by antigenic determinants (HLA) may function as an adjuvant.

Barbuto et al. used an interesting strategy for the construction of DC-based therapeutic vaccines for cancer. Healthy donor monocytes are differentiated and matured *ex vivo* and are subsequently fused to tumor cells by electrical shock, resulting in a hybrid cell. These hybrids are gamma irradiated, to prevent replication, and then administered back to the patient, seeking the generation of immune responses against neoplasms. Although the hybrids were shown to offer limited improvement of mortality rates, longer survival of the treated patients was achieved [75, 76]. Another phase I study in melanoma patients employed immunotherapy using plasmacytoid and myeloid DCs (pDC and mDC, respectively). The results were promising and indicated a survival time of more than 2 years in most of their patients [77, 78].

Currently, more than 500 clinical trials using dendritic cells are being conducted for the treatment of various forms of cancer in different countries. Most of these (324) are in the US, followed by the European Union (120) and China (72) [79]. Although results are very heterogeneous, there is a consensus that the use of these therapies in humans does not present risks or serious side effects.

Sipuleucel-T (Provenge), a dendritic cell-based vaccine for the treatment of metastatic castration-resistant prostate cancer, is the only example approved for use in humans. Its manufacture is done in a personalized manner, which involves the extraction of the patient's peripheral blood mononuclear cells (PBMCs) by leukapheresis, transport of the cells to Dendreon's facility (New Jersey, USA) for in vitro culture, maturation of DCs and loading with PA2024 (hybrid protein of GM-CSF and prostate-specific prostatic acid phosphatase, PAP) before returning the cells to the hospital where they will be administered to the patient [80].

Three phase 3 clinical trials supported the approval of sipuleucel-T by the FDA [81–83]. These studies have demonstrated that sipuleucel-T extended the survival of treated patients by 4.1 months when compared to the control group that received cells processed in a manner similar to sipuleucel-T, however, without activation due to the absence of the recombinant protein. Although this gain in survival seems promising, none of these studies showed significant increase in time to disease progression [84]. However, no side effects were observed in most cases, and T-lymphocyte proliferation was also detected, factors contributing to FDA approval [84]. In practice, the logistics of sending temperature- and time-sensitive material from widely distributed health care institutions to and from a single processing center made this immunotherapeutic strategy cumbersome and relatively expensive, since the total cost of treatment with sipuleucel-T has been reported to be $93,000 to $140,000.00 [80, 85]. Despite the prolonged survival and increased quality of life, this therapeutic option was not sustained and was discontinued.

4. Suicide gene therapy

In cancer gene therapy, different approaches can be used to kill tumor cells. Suicide gene therapy (also called gene-directed enzyme prodrug therapy) is one example where a viral or bacterial gene is introduced in the cancer cell such that it can convert a nontoxic prodrug into its lethal form. The most famous system used in this strategy is herpes simplex virus thymidine kinase gene (HSV-tk) and ganciclovir (GCV) as the prodrug. Expression of the HSV-tk gene leads to production of the enzyme that turns GCV into GCV monophosphate. After this first conversion, cellular kinases metabolize GCV monophosphate into GCV triphosphate, which is an analogue of deoxyguanosine triphosphate. GCV triphosphate causes tumor cell death upon its incorporation into DNA and consequent inhibition of DNA replication [86]. Another example of a suicide gene is the cytosine deaminase gene (CD) of *Escherichia coli* that catalyzes the hydrolytic deamination of cytosine into uracil, converting the nontoxic antifungal agent 5-fluorocytosine (5-FC) into 5-fluorouracil (5-FU). This process causes cell death by three main pathways: thymidylate synthase inhibition, formation of (5-FU) RNA and of (5-FU) DNA complexes [86]. More recent systems were developed, including an engineered version of human thymidylate kinase (TMPK) and the prodrug azidothymidine (AZT), which was first tested in leukemia model *in vitro* and *in vivo*. Native TMPK catalyzes AZT into AZT monophosphate, the toxic compound, only very slowly, so the engineering of TMPK allows it to act more robustly [87, 88]. In another example, the iCas9 system consists of inducible expression of the caspase-9 gene and administration of the small molecule chemical inducer of dimerization (CID) that leads to caspase-9 dimerization, thus promoting apoptosis [86].

One of the advantages of the suicide gene approach is the bystander effect that consists of a functional effect that may be seen even when only a small percent of cells has been transduced, and thus, tumor regression can occur. The most accepted hypotheses for this phenomenon of killing nontransduced tumor cells are passive diffusion of the drug, passage of the drug through gap junctions and release of soluble factors, forming a local bystander effect [89]. A different approach that relies on the bystander effect involves the use of mesenchymal stem cells (MSCs) to deliver drugs or vectors. The advantage in this case is that HSV-tk–modified MSCs could be effectively delivered to the area of interest and GCV could then be safely administrated systemically. HSV-tk–bearing MSCs home to and infiltrate the tumor region. Consequently, only tumor cells will be affected, while adjacent areas should remain unharmed [90].

Alternatively, the bystander effect may be a consequence of an immune response initiated by suicide gene therapy *in vivo*, also known as a distant bystander effect. Several articles in the literature have demonstrated a relationship between HSV-tk and immune response. Also called gene-mediated cytotoxic immunotherapy, treatment with HSV-tk promotes innate immune stimulation and infiltration of T cells in tumors [89]. In a clinical trial treating prostate cancer, Ayala and collaborators used an adenoviral vector encoding HSV-tk. In addition to increased apoptosis and decreased microvessel density, they found circulating and activated CD8+ cells and increased IL-12, an important mediator of immune response to tumor cells and viral infection. They also found intratumor CD8+ cells, suggesting the occurrence of both local and systemic responses [91]. Combining suicide and immune gene therapy in an aggressive melanoma model, together HSV-tk and GM-CSF induced a meaningful systemic immune response that was stronger as compared to GM-CSF alone [92]. The induction of an immune response upon CD/5-FC may be less well known [93] but has also been reported [94, 95]. Adenoviral delivery of HSV-tk was tested in a phase III trial, showing increased time to death in patients with high-grade glioma, but it did not increase overall survival [96]; perhaps combining suicide gene therapy with an additional immunotherapy approach could improve response. For example, a current trial is testing the combination of HSV-tk with FMS-like tyrosine kinase 3 ligand (FLT3L) carried by adenoviral vectors in order to promote both tumor cell death and DC activity [97].

Applied as a safety mechanism, HSV-tk is also used to control CAR-T cells. As described in more detail below, the successful clinical experience of engineered CAR-T cells is also associated with serious adverse events where the massive cell killing results in tumor lysis syndrome, an extreme elevation of plasma IL-6 concentrations that can lead to hypotension and respiratory distress in severe cases [98]. Accordingly, suicide gene therapy can be used to kill the CAR-T cells and thus stop the cytokine release syndrome [99]. In a myeloid leukemia model, Casucci and collaborators associated HSV-tk/GCV with CAR-T cells targeting the CD44v6 receptor and compared this approach with the use of the nonimmunogenic suicide gene iCas9 in an attempt to avoid an unwanted immune response, revealing that the second approach was more effective in containing the cytokine release syndrome [100]. At least three clinical trials utilizing iCas9 to control cell fate upon adoptive T cell transfer have been initiated for the treatment of leukemia and lymphoma [79, 101].

http://dx.doi.org/10.5772/intechopen.80386

In summary, suicide gene therapy is an approach that involves death mechanisms and immunotherapy. The strategy is still evolving from the initial trials and may be an interesting option against cancer and for the improved safety of CAR-T cell therapy.

5. Turning gene therapy into immunotherapy: adenovirus-carrying ARF and interferon-beta

Our own research has focused on the use of nonreplicating viral vectors for the transfer of tumor suppressor genes in combination with an immune-modulating gene (**Figure 1**). The goal is to induce both cell death and an immune response, thus overcoming the immunosuppressive tumor microenvironment and initiating the cancer immunity cycle. To this end, we have developed an improved vector system that promotes cooperation between gene function and vector performance.

We have constructed a series of viral vectors where transgene expression is controlled by the tumor suppressor p53, a powerful transcriptional regulator [54, 102, 103]. Moreover, placing the p53 cDNA under the control of the p53-responsive promoter (PGTxβ, or simply PG)

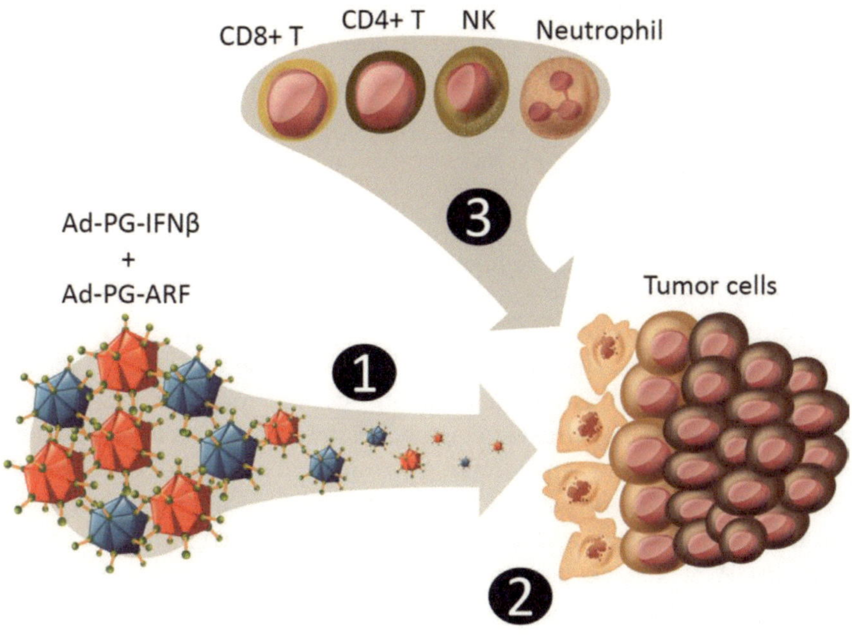

Figure 1. Schematic representation of our immunotherapy approach. (1) The adenoviral vectors encode either interferon-β (IFNβ) or p19ARF (alternate reading frame, p19ARF in mice and p14ARF in humans) where expression of the cDNA is controlled by a p53 responsive promoter, termed PG. (2) The combination of IFNβ + ARF induces tumor cell death by necroptosis and is associated with the release of immunogenic factors (such as HMGB1, ATP and calreticulin). (3) Immune cells are recruited and activated to attack the tumor.

establishes an autoregulatory, positive feedback mechanism that was shown to outperform vectors employing a constitutive promoter to express p53. That is, gene expression and cell killing *in vitro* and *in vivo* were superior when using our modified vectors to express p53 [104–106]. We have also looked to p19ARF (alternate reading frame, p19ARF in mice and p14ARF in humans), a functional partner of p53, to serve as the death-promoting factor in our approach and have observed that it is effectively expressed from our p53-responsive vectors in tumor cells that harbor wild type p53, resulting in activation of p53-mediated cell killing *in vitro* and *in vivo* [107]. Admittedly, cell killing mediated by the p53/ARF pathway alone has a limited, but recognized, role in promoting an antitumor immune response [108].

In order to activate the immune response against the tumor, we have added interferon-β (IFNβ) to our therapeutic approach since it is a central player in innate and adaptive immunity [109]. Indeed, the combination of p19Arf and IFNβ is better able to induce melanoma cell death both *in vitro* and *in vivo* [110, 111]. Strikingly, the mechanism of cell death involves necroptosis with liberation of the classic markers of immunogenic cell death [111]. In a mouse model of melanoma, we have confirmed the induction of an antitumor immune response in vaccine and immunotherapy settings, with critical involvement of NK cells, CD4+ and CD8+ T cells [112]. In a mouse model of lung carcinoma, we have shown that *in situ* gene therapy can bring about an antitumor immune response with critical involvement of neutrophils [113]. Together these studies show that our gene transfer approach is an effective immunotherapy [114, 115]. The results to date are promising and research will continue to evolve, with critical development using clinically relevant models, such as testing with patient-derived tumor samples as well as alternative animal models, including canines [116].

6. Oncolytic virotherapy

In 1892, viruses were first noted by humans and it took only a few years for researchers to raise the possibility that some viral infections may interfere in the clinical outcomes of some patients with different types of cancers. In 1904, a transitory spontaneous remission of acute leukemia in a patient after infection with influenza was reported, prompting the observation of additional occurrences of this type and paving the way for the concept of virotherapy [117]. One of the first reports of viruses being deliberately applied as a therapeutic approach for cancer dates back to 1949, when Herman A. Hoster and colleagues evaluated the clinical outcome of 21 Hodgkin's disease patients after intentional exposure to Hepatitis B virus [118]. Some years after that, Newman and Southam evaluated the use of several different viruses (vaccinia, mumps, West Nile, dengue, among others) for the treatment of advanced cancer in 57 patients, though no remarkable clinical outcome was observed [119].

Concomitant with the expansion of knowledge in the field of virology, additional protocols describing novel attempts to establish cancer virotherapy were reported, including the use of an array of different virus species, such as adenovirus, Coxsackie, and Epstein-Barr. Despite the new investigations in the 1970s, the threshold of "transitory response" could not be surpassed due to adverse events, such as neurotoxicity, possibly associated with technological limits related to the handling of viruses, for example, the lack of genetic engineering tools needed for the development and testing of more effective and safer versions [120].

With the advances in molecular and cellular biology as well as animal models for cancer research, the perspective of taking oncolytic virotherapy (OV) from bench to the bedside became feasible. For example, a report in 1991 described the construction of a modified herpes simplex virus (HSV-1), which was thymidine kinase-negative and attenuated for neurotoxicity [121]; thus, a critical step was taken to advance the technology of OV.

By definition, OV encompasses native or genetically engineered viruses whose replication is restricted to tumor cells. As per the immunotherapy trend, OV is increasingly gaining attention due to its performance in clinical trials where it is used to treat several types of cancers. With the 2015 approval of Imlygic (talimogene laherparepvec, OncoVex, T-VEC, an HSV-based oncolytic virus) by the FDA and the EMA (European Medicines Agency) for the treatment of unresectable melanoma, the principle of taking advantage of viral replication in order to treat cancer is now an established therapeutic approach.

6.1. Targeting and mechanism of OV

Even in the absence of tools to genetically modify viruses in order to make them safer, in the 1950s, Alice Moore observed that it was possible to generate virus strains with higher oncolytic capacity and more tumor specificity through adaptation. In particular, the oncolytic features of Russian encephalitis virus were enhanced after 20–30 passages in the Sarcoma 180 cell line as compared to the original strain, leading to the idea that the tumor cells could exert an evolutionary pressure upon the virus, favoring those particles adapted to replicate in the tumor [122].

After the development of techniques for the manipulation of DNA, these tools were used to break down the barriers for the development of virotherapy. Thus, undesirable virulence could be mitigated by eliminating key genes from the viral genome, generating attenuated viruses. The viral genome often codes important proteins that regulate its replication in post-mitotic cells. For example, the thymidine kinase (TK) gene is associated with DNA synthesis and cell cycle progression [123]. Taking advantage of this information, Martuza and collaborators showed that HSV lacking the gene coding for TK could replicate in dividing cells, but replication was hampered in quiescent cells, in line with the need for selective replication in tumor cells. In an animal model of glioma, locally administrated mutant HSV led to inhibition of tumor growth and showed decreased neurotoxicity [121]. Alternatively, the viral life cycle may be guided by cellular or virus-encoded microRNAs that alter the level of expression of cell-specific proteins [124].

In addition to the aforementioned approaches, tumor selectivity may be achieved by directing the interactions between the virus particle and the target cell. The retargeting of the viral particles can be achieved in different ways, such as the genetic modification of viral proteins so that they gain specificity for a particular cell surface protein. Alternatively, the use of bispecific adapters mediates the interaction of native capsid proteins with a specific cellular receptor. The virus may also be detargeted, that is, modified so that it no longer interacts with nontumor cells [125].

Besides the transductional targeting, the tropism can be also altered at the transcriptional level by using a tissue-specific promoter to regulate the expression of genes critical for viral replication. As an example, in order to produce adenovirus whose replication is restricted to prostate cancer cells, expression of the *E1A* adenoviral gene (essential for regulating adenoviral replication) was placed under the control of the prostate-specific antigen (PSA) promoter, leading to an adenovirus that is only able to replicate in prostate cells [126].

Viruses themselves are entities capable of subverting the cell replication machinery and making a favorable environment for their own replication, which occasionally leads to cell death by lysis when the new viral particles are released and the infection cycle continues, increasing the initial quantity of viral particles that is then only limited by the decreased number of target cell as well as by the direct action of the immune system through an antiviral response. In addition to lysis due to viral replication, some viruses can produce proteins that trigger molecular pathways that lead to cell death, as is the case for adenovirus, whose E3-11.6 K transcript is found to be important for the lysis of infected cells [127, 128]. However, more recently, it was found that the immune system, concomitant to the intrinsic effect of oncolytic infection, plays an important role.

After infection, more precisely after cell lysis, the release of intracellular content participates in the activation of both innate and adaptive immune responses against tumor- and virus-associated antigens, potentially reverting the intrinsic immune tolerance of the tumor microenvironment [129]. After rupture of the cellular membrane by the virions, the following release of PAMPs and DAMPs induces the activation of type I interferon, Toll-like receptor–mediated molecular pathways and the production of cytokines, which culminate in the recruitment and activation of antigen-presenting cells (APCs) and the subsequent establishment of a memory immune response [130].

6.2. Oncolytic virotherapy makes its mark: oncolytics with regulatory approval for the treatment of cancer

In 2005, Oncorine (H101, Onyx-015), an adenovirus-based oncolytic developed by Shanghai Sunway Biotech, was approved by State Food and Drug Administration, China (SFDA), for the treatment of head and neck squamous cell carcinoma [131]. Oncorine is a modified adenovirus whose E1B and E3 genes are deleted, leading to a virus that, it was originally thought, should only replicate in cells that lack p53 activity, mainly tumor cells [132, 133], though other mechanisms have been proposed for Oncorine's tumor selectivity [134]. Its precursor, Onyx-15, showed good performance in clinical trials, especially when combined with additional therapeutic approaches, and was well tolerated and safe [135], with no therapy-associated severe adverse events when administered intratumorally in gliomas [136]. In addition to its safety profile, Onyx-15 administration may be associated with some clinical improvement for patients with metastatic colorectal cancer who failed the first-line therapy [137] and those with hepatobiliary tumors not eligible for surgical resection [138].

In 2015, the FDA and the EMA approved an OV based on a modified herpes simplex virus (HSV-1) for the treatment of melanoma. Imlygic (OncoVex, T-VEC, talimogene laherparepvec) expresses granulocyte-macrophage colony-stimulating factor (GM-CSF), while viral genes ICP34.5 and ICP47 were deleted, modifications that conferred better replication in tumor cells and stimulation of an antitumor immune response [30]. After showing safety and antitumor activity in experimental models [30], Imlygic was then administered in a phase I clinical trial, in patients with cutaneous or subcutaneous metastases from refractory head and neck carcinoma, melanoma, breast and gastrointestinal adenocarcinoma, being well tolerated and provoking only mild adverse events (local erythema and fever) [139]. Encouraged by these results, efficacy was assessed in a phase II clinical trial carried out with 50 stages III and IV melanoma patients. In this study, mild adverse events were observed and there was a 26% Response Evaluation Criteria in Solid Tumors (RECIST) response rate, including 8 complete and 5 partial responses [140]. Based on these positive results, an open-label phase III study was carried out where therapy with Imlygic was compared to treatment with GM-CSF, revealing high tolerance to the treatment, and a higher durable response rate (DRR) and also overall survival compared to the GM-CSF treatment, results that culminated in the first FDA and EMA approval of an OV [141].

7. CAR-T cells

An emerging and exciting subject in cellular therapies relies on the engineering of cytotoxic T cells and natural killer cells so they can recognize specific antigens on the cell membrane and induce cell death without reliance on MHC or costimulator expression. Even though infiltrating T cells may recognize tumor antigens, they may be unable to induce a cytotoxic response due to a strong inhibitory microenvironment [142]. The modification of patients' T cells to express a chimeric antigen receptor (CAR) creates the opportunity to induce a strong cytotoxic response against the tumor even in the face of negative signals [143].

Transmembrane CAR receptors have two main functions: the first is to recognize a specific antigen present only in the membrane of tumor cells. The second is to induce signal transduction independently of other costimulatory signals, culminating in the release of cytotoxic signals and T cell proliferation [144]. Physiologically, the activation of a cytotoxic T cell is mediated by a T cell receptor (TCR) in an MHC-dependent context. Though this antigen-receptor interaction is insufficient to bring about cell killing, it is imperative that other transmembrane receptors interact, authorizing T cells to exert their cytotoxic function. Moreover, the tumor has several mechanisms to evade T cell responses, from losing the MHC complex to expressing inhibitory molecules that induce T cell exhaustion and anergy. Therefore, modifying the TCR so they do not depend upon other authorizing signals has proven an exciting strategy [142].

Structurally, a CAR has an extracellular component responsible for recognizing the antigen of interest, comprised of a single-chain variable fragment (scFv), followed by a spacer region whose length may vary, a transmembrane region (TM), and an intracellular domain composed of one or more signaling components associated with T cell activation. The first generation included, on the intracellular domain, the ζ-chain, a portion of the T cell receptor responsible for its activity. Improved understanding of the complementary signals needed for activation lead to the development of second-generation CARs, which include a CD28 costimulatory domain, thus ensuring full activation of the T cell. The third generation included other transduction signaling domains, preferentially originating from transmembrane proteins derived from the TNF superfamily, such as CD27, 4-1BB and OX40. All of them can transduce signals resulting in survival, proliferation and maintenance of T cells. The fourth generation uses a vector to deliver, in addition to CAR, cytokine genes, such as IL-2 or IL-12, whose expression changes the tumor microenvironment in favor of T cell activity [144].

The first insight into the development of a chimeric transmembrane receptor that could activate cytotoxic T cells came in 1989 by Gross and colleagues. And in 2017, the FDA approved the first two CAR-T cell therapies in rapid succession. These CARs target CD19, a molecule expressed only in B-lymphocytes, an approach shown to be a powerful second-line treatment against B cell acute lymphoblastic leukemia (B-ALL) (Kymriah—tisagenlecleucel, August 2017 [145]) and certain B cell lymphomas (Yescarta—axicabtagene ciloleucel, September 2017 [146]). While both present a scFv against CD19, Kymriah uses the 4-1BB whereas Yescarta uses CD28 as costimulatory domains. The success in clinical trials ranged from 70 to 94%, making these treatments a breakthrough in gene and immunotherapy [144]. However, there are cytotoxic effects that in some cases can be intense, caused by the killing of large numbers of cancer cells that release cytokines and waste products, leading to harmful consequences in the patients. Thus, much more is needed to understand and manage the side effects of these new and promising therapies, such as the inclusion of a suicide gene to eliminate overactive CAR-T cells [147].

Despite the incredible potential of this therapeutic strategy, CAR-T cells have some limitations that prevent their effective use in the fight against a wide range of tumors. Among them, the most troubling is the lack of a perfect antigen present only in tumor cells but not in other tissues. Tandem CAR and inhibitory chimeric antigen receptors (iCAR) are some of the strategies with the greatest potential to overcome this barrier. Tandem CAR consists of two chimeric receptors designed to provide costimulatory signals in response to the recognition of two different antigens [144]. Only after the recognition of both signals are the tandem CAR cells activated. On the other hand, iCAR aims to inhibit T cell activity as soon as the second specific antigen is recognized [144].This second antigen does not exist in tumor cells, so when the iCAR-T cells find it, they are inhibited and leave nontumor cells unscathed.

In some studies, the inhibitory molecules used in the construction of iCAR-T cells are derived from the intracellular domains of proteins often expressed by tumors and whose function is to evade the immune system. Well-known examples are the receptors CTLA-4 and PD-1 that reduce the potency of TCR signaling. The fusion of their intracellular domain to a CAR also inhibits signaling, resulting in decreased cytokine production, limited lymphocyte motility and reduced target cell lysis [144].

Another hindrance to the application of CAR cell therapies is their large-scale production. The usual steps to produce CAR cells are based on extraction of cells from the patient, genetic engineering of NK or T cells, expansion and infusion in the patient. Due to the laborious process, few health care institutions are prepared to produce CAR cells. And off-site preparation of the CAR cells presents extensive logistical challenges. Thus, the production of the CAR cells is one of the principle factors that promote the high cost of this therapy. In a remarkable research conducted by Smith and colleagues [148], they have developed an approach that may show a way around this problem. In a mouse model, they have modified the circulating T cells within the animal's own body. The strategy is based on the transfection of the CAR gene using β-amino-ester–based nanoparticles. For this, nanocarriers were coated with CD3, a lymphocyte surface antigen. The recognition of this antigen induces the endocytosis of the nanocarriers by the lymphocytes. Furthermore, peptides containing microtubule-associated sequences (MTAS) and nuclear localization signals (NLS) were added to the polymer, facilitating the rapid import of its genetic load through microtubule transport machinery. Alternative approaches include the use of viral vectors and the use of transposon/transposase systems, such as sleeping beauty, that promote integration of the CAR sequence in the host DNA [148].

Instead of a complicated scenario of transporting of patients' cells to and from specialized facilities, methodology enabling *in situ* modification of T cells implies that nanoparticles, virus and other vectors containing the CAR sequence can be produced in a central location, packaged and shipped to any hospital. All that is needed is a syringe to inject the vector into the bloodstream of the patient. As the nanoparticles are stable, this enables long-term storage, reducing the cost of this medical technology and permitting the sale of CAR cell therapies at more affordable prices.

8. Conclusions

Clearly, cancer immunotherapy can be achieved by a variety of interventions that share the common goal of boosting the antitumor immune response. These modalities may target distinct points along the cancer immunity cycle, from inducing immunogenic cell death, promoting antigen presentation and culminating in activation of innate and adaptive responses, including cytolytic T cell activity, which can then further promote antitumor immunity since tumor cell killing would reinitiate and propagate the cycle [149]. Moreover, distinct points in the cancer immunity cycle may be targeted simultaneously, enhancing even more the antitumor response.

As shown here, gene transfer plays a critical role in several key cancer immunotherapies. Vaccines, suicide gene therapy, simultaneous induction of cell death and immune response, OV and CAR-T cells all benefit from gene transfer. While the gene transfer technology will continue to evolve, the therapeutic benefit of genetically modifying cells in order to alter their function will certainly continue to be a central theme in cancer immunotherapy. The approval of Imlygic (FDA and EMA), Yescarta and Kymriah (FDA and EMA), as well as the commercialization of Oncorine (China) show that immunotherapies involving some component of gene transfer are now well established.

In addition, we expect that future approaches will rely on multiple immunotherapies that work in harmony. For example, checkpoint blockade along with the gene transfer interventions should bring about strategic combinations of inducing cell death, tumor-specific immune response and maintenance of cytolytic T cell activity. Challenges remain to be addressed, such as avoiding adverse effects, proper monitoring criteria, identification of adequate biomarkers and definition of a reasonable price tag for cutting edge, personalized interventions. Thus, immunotherapies require further study. As such future developments unfold, gene transfer technologies are expected to remain as crucial components of cancer immunotherapy.

Acknowledgements

We are grateful for the funding that supported this effort, including the Sao Paulo Research Foundation (FAPESP, grant 15/26580-9 and fellowships 13/16074-3, PRDV; 16/18197-3, ILV; 17/23068-0, OLDC; 17/25284-2, OAR) and the National Council of Scientific and Technical Development (CNPq, fellowship 302888/2017-9, BES).

Conflict of interest

The authors have no conflicts of interest.

Author details

Otto L.D. Cerqueira, Gissele Rolemberg Oliveira Silva, Igor de Luna Vieira, Marlous Vinícius Gomes Lana, Nadine Gimenez, Otavio Augusto Rodrigues, Paulo Roberto Del Valle, Samir Andrade Mendonça and Bryan E. Strauss*

*Address all correspondence to: bstrauss@usp.br

Viral Vector Laboratory, Center for Translational Investigation in Oncology/LIM24, Cancer Institute of São Paulo, School of Medicine, University of São Paulo, Brazil

References

[1] Ehrlich P. Uber den jetzigen Stand der Karzinomforschung. Nederlands Tijdschrift voor Geneeskunde. 1909;**5**:273-290

[2] Burnet F. The Concept of Immunological Surveillance. Oxford, UK: Pergamon Press; 1970

[3] Thomas L. On immunosurveillance in human cancer. The Yale Journal of Biology and Medicine. 1982;**55**(3-4):329

[4] Hanahan D, Weinberg RA. Hallmarks of cancer: The next generation. Cell. 2011;**144**(5): 646-674

[5] Dunn GP, Old LJ, Schreiber RD. The immunobiology of cancer immunosurveillance and immunoediting. Immunity. 2004;**21**(2):137-148

[6] Teng MW, Galon J, Fridman W-H, Smyth MJ. From mice to humans: Developments in cancer immunoediting. Journal of Clinical Investigation. 2015;**125**(9):3338

[7] Zitvogel L, Tesniere A, Kroemer G. Cancer despite immunosurveillance: Immunoselection and immunosubversion. Nature Reviews Immunology. 2006;**6**(10):715-727

[8] Shankaran V, Ikeda H, Bruce AT, White JM, Swanson PE, Old LJ, et al. IFNgamma and lymphocytes prevent primary tumour development and shape tumour immunogenicity. Nature. Apr 26, 2001;**410**(6832):1107-1111

[9] Alexandrov LB, Nik-Zainal S, Wedge DC, Aparicio SA, Behjati S, Biankin AV, et al. Signatures of mutational processes in human cancer. Nature. 2013;**500**(7463):415

[10] Van Den Eynde BJ, van der Bruggen P. T cell defined tumor antigens. Current Opinion in Immunology. 1997;**9**(5):684-693

[11] Dunn GP, Old LJ, Schreiber RD. The three Es of cancer immunoediting. Annual Review of Immunology. 2004;**22**:329-360

[12] Marcus A, Gowen BG, Thompson TW, Iannello A, Ardolino M, Deng W, et al. Recognition of tumors by the innate immune system and natural killer cells. Advances in Immunology. 2014;**122**:91-128

[13] Curiel TJ. Tregs and rethinking cancer immunotherapy. Journal of Clinical Investigation. 2007;**117**(5):1167

[14] Platten M, Wick W. Tregs in gliomas—The jury is still out. Neuro-Oncology. 2015;**17**(6): 769-770. DOI: 10.1093/neuonc/nov034

[15] Ramos RN, Moraes CJD, Zelante B, Barbuto JAM. What are the molecules involved in regulatory T-cells induction by dendritic cells in cancer? Clinical and Developmental Immunology. 2013;**2013**:e806025

[16] Valentini AM, Di Pinto F, Cariola F, Guerra V, Giannelli G, Caruso ML, et al. PD-L1 expression in colorectal cancer defines three subsets of tumor immune microenvironments. Oncotarget. Feb 2018;**9**(9):8584-8596

[17] Yu DP, Cheng X, Liu ZD, Xu SF. Comparative beneficiary effects of immunotherapy against chemotherapy in patients with advanced NSCLC: Meta-analysis and systematic review. Oncology Letters. Aug 2017;**14**(2):1568-1580

[18] Mellman I, Coukos G, Dranoff G. Cancer immunotherapy comes of age. Nature. Dec 2011;**480**(7378):480-489

[19] Nahta R, Esteva FJ. Herceptin: Mechanisms of action and resistance. Cancer Letters. Feb 2006;**232**(2):123-138

[20] Trinh VA, Joseph J, Hwu WJ. Anti-programmed cell death-1 (PD-1) monoclonal antibodies in treating advanced melanoma—A clinical update. Discovery Medicine. Jan 2018;**25**(135):31-40

[21] Larkin J, Hodi FS, Wolchok JD. Combined nivolumab and ipilimumab or monotherapy in untreated melanoma. The New England Journal of Medicine. Sep 2015;**373**(13): 1270-1271

[22] Ali OA, Lewin SA, Dranoff G, Mooney DJ. Vaccines combined with immune checkpoint antibodies promote cytotoxic T-cell activity and tumor eradication. Cancer Immunology Research. Feb 2016;**4**(2):95-100

[23] Duraiswamy J, Freeman GJ, Coukos G. Dual blockade of PD-1 and CTLA-4 combined with tumor vaccine effectively restores T-cell rejection function in tumors--response. Cancer Research. Jan 2014;**74**(2):633-634; discussion 5

[24] Bourgeois-Daigneault MC, Roy DG, Aitken AS, El Sayes N, Martin NT, Varette O, et al. Neoadjuvant oncolytic virotherapy before surgery sensitizes triple-negative breast cancer to immune checkpoint therapy. Science Translational Medicine. Jan 3, 2018;**10**(422):eaao1641

[25] Samson A, Scott KJ, Taggart D, West EJ, Wilson E, Nuovo GJ, et al. Intravenous delivery of oncolytic reovirus to brain tumor patients immunologically primes for subsequent checkpoint blockade. Science Translational Medicine. Jan 3, 2018;**10**(422):eaam7577

[26] Smith BD, Kasamon YL, Kowalski J, Gocke C, Murphy K, Miller CB, et al. K562/GM-CSF immunotherapy reduces tumor burden in chronic myeloid leukemia patients with residual disease on imatinib mesylate. Clinical Cancer Research. Jan 2010;**16**(1):338-347

[27] Lipson EJ, Sharfman WH, Chen S, McMiller TL, Pritchard TS, Salas JT, et al. Safety and immunologic correlates of melanoma GVAX, a GM-CSF secreting allogeneic melanoma cell vaccine administered in the adjuvant setting. Journal of Translational Medicine. Jul 2015;**13**:214

[28] Lutz E, Yeo CJ, Lillemoe KD, Biedrzycki B, Kobrin B, Herman J, et al. A lethally irradiated allogeneic granulocyte-macrophage colony stimulating factor-secreting tumor vaccine for pancreatic adenocarcinoma. A phase II trial of safety, efficacy, and immune activation. Annals of Surgery. Feb 2011;**253**(2):328-335

[29] Simons JW, Sacks N. Granulocyte-macrophage colony-stimulating factor-transduced allogeneic cancer cellular immunotherapy: The GVAX vaccine for prostate cancer. Urologic Oncology. Sep–Oct 2006;**24**(5):419-424

[30] Liu BL, Robinson M, Han ZQ, Branston RH, English C, Reay P, et al. ICP34.5 deleted herpes simplex virus with enhanced oncolytic, immune stimulating, and anti-tumour properties. Gene Therapy. Feb 2003;**10**(4):292-303

[31] Guillerey C, Huntington ND, Smyth MJ. Targeting natural killer cells in cancer immunotherapy. Nature Immunology. Aug 2016;**17**(9):1025-1036

[32] Ramos CA, Dotti G. Chimeric antigen receptor (CAR)-engineered lymphocytes for cancer therapy. Expert Opinion on Biological Therapy. Jul 2011;**11**(7):855-873

[33] Park JH, Rivière I, Gonen M, Wang X, Sénéchal B, Curran KJ, et al. Long-term follow-up of CD19 CAR therapy in acute lymphoblastic leukemia. New England Journal of Medicine. Feb 2018;**378**(5):449-459

[34] Turtle CJ, Hay KA, Hanafi LA, Li D, Cherian S, Chen X, et al. Durable molecular remissions in chronic lymphocytic leukemia treated with CD19-specific chimeric antigen receptor-modified T cells after failure of Ibrutinib. Journal of Clinical Oncology. Sep 2017;**35**(26):3010-3020

[35] Quintás-Cardama A. CAR T-cell therapy in large B-cell lymphoma. New England Journal of Medicine. Mar 2018;**378**(11):1065

[36] Yoon DH, Osborn MJ, Tolar J, Kim CJ. Incorporation of immune checkpoint blockade into chimeric antigen receptor T cells (CAR-Ts): Combination or built-in CAR-T. International Journal of Molecular Sciences. Jan 2018;**19**(2):e340

[37] Carreno BM, Magrini V, Becker-Hapak M, Kaabinejadian S, Hundal J, Petti AA, et al. Cancer immunotherapy. A dendritic cell vaccine increases the breadth and diversity of melanoma neoantigen-specific T cells. Science. May 15, 2015;**348**(6236):803-808

[38] Steinman RM, Mellman I. Immunotherapy: Bewitched, bothered, and bewildered no more. Science. Jul 9, 2004;**305**(5681):197-200

[39] Coley WB. The treatment of malignant tumors by repeated inoculations of erysipelas: With a report of ten original cases. The American Journal of the Medical Sciences. 1893;**5**:487-511

[40] Lamm DL, Thor DE, Harris SC, Reyna JA, Stogdill VD, Radwin HM. Bacillus Calmette-Guerin immunotherapy of superficial bladder cancer. The Journal of urology. Jul 1980;**124**(1):38-40

[41] O'Hagan DT, Valiante NM. Recent advances in the discovery and delivery of vaccine adjuvants. Nature Reviews. Drug Discovery. Sep 2003;**2**(9):727-735

[42] O'Hagan DT, MacKichan ML, Singh M. Recent developments in adjuvants for vaccines against infectious diseases. Biomolecular Engineering. 2001;**18**(3):69-85

[43] Lima KM, dos Santos SA, Rodrigues JM Jr, Silva CL. Vaccine adjuvant: It makes the difference. Vaccine. 2004;**22**(19):2374-2379

[44] Takeda K, Akira S. TLR signaling pathways. Seminars in Immunology. Feb 2004;**16**(1):3-9

[45] Inohara C, McDonald C, Nunez G. NOD-LRR proteins: Role in host-microbial interactions and inflammatory disease. Annual Review of Biochemistry. 2005;**74**:355-383

[46] Delneste Y, Beauvillain C, Jeannin P. Innate immunity: Structure and function of TLRs. Medecine Sciences. Jan 2007;**23**(1):67-73

[47] Takeda K, Akira S. Toll-like receptors in innate immunity. International Immunology. Jan 2005;**17**(1):1-14

[48] Trinchieri G, Sher A. Cooperation of toll-like receptor signals in innate immune defence. Nature Reviews. Immunology. Mar 2007;**7**(3):179-190

[49] Kash N, Lee MA, Kollipara R, Downing C, Guidry J, Tyring SK. Safety and efficacy data on vaccines and immunization to human papillomavirus. Journal of Clinical Medicine. Apr 3, 2015;**4**(4):614-633

[50] Rosenberg SA, Yang JC, Schwartzentruber DJ, Hwu P, Marincola FM, Topalian SL, et al. Immunologic and therapeutic evaluation of a synthetic peptide vaccine for the treatment of patients with metastatic melanoma. Nature Medicine. Mar 1998;**4**(3):321-327

[51] Butts C, Socinski MA, Mitchell PL, Thatcher N, Havel L, Krzakowski M, et al. Tecemotide (L-BLP25) versus placebo after chemoradiotherapy for stage III non-small-cell lung cancer (START): A randomised, double-blind, phase 3 trial. The Lancet Oncology. Jan 2014;**15**(1):59-68

[52] Robinson HL, Pertmer TM. DNA vaccines for viral infections: Basic studies and applications. Advances in Virus Research. 2000;**55**:1-74

[53] Panicali D, Davis SW, Weinberg RL, Paoletti E. Construction of live vaccines by using genetically engineered poxviruses: Biological activity of recombinant vaccinia virus expressing influenza virus hemagglutinin. Proceedings of the National Academy of Sciences. 1983;**80**(17):5364-5368

[54] Bajgelman MC, Strauss BE. Development of an adenoviral vector with robust expression driven by p53. Virology. Feb 5, 2008;**371**(1):8-13

[55] Valdmanis PN, Lisowski L, Kay MA. rAAV-mediated tumorigenesis: Still unresolved after an AAV assault. Molecular Therapy. Nov 2012;**20**(11):2014-2017

[56] Fukuhara H, Ino Y, Todo T. Oncolytic virus therapy: A new era of cancer treatment at dawn. Cancer Science. Oct 2016;**107**(10):1373-1379

[57] Ledford H. Engineered cell therapy for cancer gets thumbs up from FDA advisers. Nature. Jul 12, 2017;**547**(7663):270

[58] Monaco L, Faccio L. Patient-driven search for rare disease therapies: The Fondazione Telethon success story and the strategy leading to Strimvelis. EMBO Molecular Medicine. Mar 2017;**9**(3):289-292

[59] FDA. FDA Approves Novel Gene Therapy to Treat Patients with a Rare Form of Inherited Vision Loss. FDA, Silver, Spring: MD, USA; Available from: https://www.fda.gov/NewsEvents/Newsroom/PressAnnouncements/ucm589467.htm

[60] Ott PA, Hodi FS, Kaufman HL, Wigginton JM, Wolchok JD. Combination immunotherapy: A road map. Journal for Immunotherapy of Cancer. 2017;**5**:16

[61] Mahoney KM, Rennert PD, Freeman GJ. Combination cancer immunotherapy and new immunomodulatory targets. Nature Reviews. Drug Discovery. Aug 2015;**14**(8):561-584

[62] Versteven M, Van den Bergh JMJ, Marcq E, Smits ELJ, Van Tendeloo VFI, Hobo W, et al. Dendritic cells and programmed death-1 blockade: A joint venture to combat cancer. Frontiers in Immunology. 2018;**9**:394

[63] Vazquez-Lombardi R, Roome B, Christ D. Molecular engineering of therapeutic cytokines. Antibodies. 2013;**2**(3):426-451

[64] Dranoff G. Cytokines in cancer pathogenesis and cancer therapy. Nature Reviews Cancer. Jan 2004;**4**(1):11-22

[65] Baldo BA. Side effects of cytokines approved for therapy. Drug Safety. Nov 2014;**37**(11):921-943

[66] Syn NL, Teng MWL, Mok TSK, Soo RA. De-novo and acquired resistance to immune checkpoint targeting. The Lancet Oncology. Dec 2017;**18**(12):e731-ee41

[67] Cameron F, Whiteside G, Perry C. Ipilimumab: First global approval. Drugs. May 28, 2011;**71**(8):1093-1104

[68] Pardoll DM. The blockade of immune checkpoints in cancer immunotherapy. Nature reviews Cancer. Mar 22, 2012;**12**(4):252-264

[69] Guermonprez P, Valladeau J, Zitvogel L, Théry C, Amigorena S. Antigen presentation and T cell stimulation by dendritic cells. Annual Review of Immunology. 2002;**20**(1):621-667

[70] Fernandez NC, Lozier A, Flament C, Ricciardi-Castagnoli P, Bellet D, Suter M, et al. Dendritic cells directly trigger NK cell functions: Cross-talk relevant in innate antitumor immune responses in vivo. Nature Medicine. 1999;**5**(4):405-411

[71] Kinsey GR, Okusa MD. Expanding role of T cells in acute kidney injury. Current Opinion in Nephrology and Hypertension. 2014;**23**(1):9

[72] Pinho MP, Bergami-Santos PC, Barbuto JAM. T cell stimulation by dendritic cell-tumor cell hybrids is enhanced in the presence of free dendritic cells. Journal for Immunotherapy of Cancer. 2013;**1**(1):1

[73] Palucka K, Banchereau J. Dendritic cell-based cancer therapeutic vaccines. Immunity. Jul 25, 2013;**39**(1):38-48

[74] Romagnoli GG, Zelante BB, Toniolo PA, Migliori IK, Barbuto JAM. Dendritic cell-derived exosomes may be a tool for cancer immunotherapy by converting tumor cells into immunogenic targets. Frontiers in Immunology. 2015;**5**:692

[75] Barbuto JAM, Ensina LF, Neves AR, Bergami-Santos PC, Leite KR, Marques R, et al. Dendritic cell-tumor cell hybrid vaccination for metastatic cancer. Cancer Immunology, Immunotherapy. 2004;**53**(12):1111-1118

[76] Pinho MP, Sundarasetty BS, Bergami-Santos PC, Steponavicius-Cruz K, Ferreira AK, Stripecke R, et al. Dendritic-tumor cell hybrids induce tumor-specific immune responses more effectively than the simple mixture of dendritic and tumor cells. Cytotherapy. 2016;**18**(4):570-580

[77] Schreibelt G, Bol KF, Westdorp H, Wimmers F, Aarntzen EH, Duiveman-de Boer T, et al. Effective clinical responses in metastatic melanoma patients after vaccination with primary myeloid dendritic cells. Clinical Cancer Research. May 1, 2016;**22**(9):2155-2166

[78] Bol KF, Schreibelt G, Gerritsen WR, de Vries IJ, Figdor CG. Dendritic cell-based immunotherapy: State of the art and beyond. Clinical Cancer Research. Apr 15, 2016;**22**(8):1897-1906

[79] NIH. April 2018. Available from: https://www.clinicaltrials.gov/ct2/home

[80] Graff JN, Chamberlain ED. Sipuleucel-T in the treatment of prostate cancer: An evidence-based review of its place in therapy. Core Evidence. 2015;**10**:1-10

[81] Kantoff PW, Higano CS, Shore ND, Berger ER, Small EJ, Penson DF, et al. Sipuleucel-T immunotherapy for castration-resistant prostate cancer. New England Journal of Medicine. 2010;**363**(5):411-422

[82] Small EJ, Schellhammer PF, Higano CS, Redfern CH, Nemunaitis JJ, Valone FH, et al. Placebo-controlled phase III trial of immunologic therapy with sipuleucel-T (APC8015) in patients with metastatic, asymptomatic hormone refractory prostate cancer. Journal of Clinical Oncology. 2006;**24**(19):3089-3094

[83] Higano CS, Schellhammer PF, Small EJ, Burch PA, Nemunaitis J, Yuh L, et al. Integrated data from 2 randomized, double-blind, placebo-controlled, phase 3 trials of active cellular immunotherapy with sipuleucel-T in advanced prostate cancer. Cancer. 2009;**115**(16): 3670-3679

[84] Anassi E, Ndefo UA. Sipuleucel-T (provenge) injection: The first immunotherapy agent (vaccine) for hormone-refractory prostate cancer. Pharmacy and Therapeutics. Apr 2011;**36**(4):197-202

[85] Miller D. Dendreon's Provenge Costs the Same as Chemotherapy. Minyanville; 2010. Available from: http://www.minyanville.com/businessmarkets/articles/dendreon-provenge-cost-taxotere-sanofi-aventis/7/29/2010/id/29371 [Accessed: Jun 2018]

[86] Duarte S, Carle G, Faneca H, de Lima MC, Pierrefite-Carle V. Suicide gene therapy in cancer: Where do we stand now? Cancer Letters. Nov 28, 2012;**324**(2):160-170

[87] Sato T, Neschadim A, Lavie A, Yanagisawa T, Medin JA. The engineered thymidylate kinase (TMPK)/AZT enzyme-prodrug axis offers efficient bystander cell killing for suicide gene therapy of cancer. PLoS One. 2013;**8**(10):e78711

[88] Sato T, Neschadim A, Konrad M, Fowler DH, Lavie A, Medin JA. Engineered human tmpk/AZT as a novel enzyme/prodrug axis for suicide gene therapy. Molecular Therapy: The Journal of the American Society of Gene Therapy. May 2007;**15**(5):962-970

[89] Aguilar LK, Guzik BW, Aguilar-Cordova E. Cytotoxic immunotherapy strategies for cancer: Mechanisms and clinical development. Journal of Cellular Biochemistry. Aug 2011;**112**(8):1969-1977

[90] Nowakowski A, Drela K, Rozycka J, Janowski M, Lukomska B. Engineered mesenchymal stem cells as an anti-cancer trojan horse. Stem Cells and Development. Oct 2016;**25**(20): 1513-1531

[91] Ayala G, Satoh T, Li R, Shalev M, Gdor Y, Aguilar-Cordova E, et al. Biological response determinants in HSV-tk + ganciclovir gene therapy for prostate cancer. Molecular Therapy: The Journal of the American Society of Gene Therapy. Apr 2006;**13**(4):716-728

[92] Villaverde MS, Combe K, Duchene AG, Wei MX, Glikin GC, Finocchiaro LM. Suicide plus immune gene therapy prevents post-surgical local relapse and increases overall

survival in an aggressive mouse melanoma setting. International Immunopharmacology. Sep 2014;**22**(1):167-175

[93] Eisold S, Antolovic D, Schmidt J, Wiessner R, Klar E, von Knebel-Doeberitz M, et al. Effective antitumoral immune responses are not induced by cytosine deaminase suicide gene transfer in a syngeneic rat pancreatic carcinoma model. European Surgical Research. 2006;**38**(6):513-521

[94] Cloughesy TF, Landolfi J, Hogan DJ, Bloomfield S, Carter B, Chen CC, et al. Phase 1 trial of vocimagene amiretrorepvec and 5-fluorocytosine for recurrent high-grade glioma. Science Translational Medicine. Jun 1, 2016;**8**(341):341ra75

[95] Yagiz K, Rodriguez-Aguirre ME, Lopez Espinoza F, Montellano TT, Mendoza D, Mitchell LA, et al. A retroviral replicating vector encoding cytosine deaminase and 5-FC induces immune memory in metastatic colorectal cancer models. Molecular Therapy—Oncolytics. Mar 30, 2018;**8**:14-26

[96] Westphal M, Yla-Herttuala S, Martin J, Warnke P, Menei P, Eckland D, et al. Adenovirus-mediated gene therapy with sitimagene ceradenovec followed by intravenous ganciclovir for patients with operable high-grade glioma (ASPECT): A randomised, open-label, phase 3 trial. The Lancet Oncology. Aug 2013;**14**(9):823-833

[97] Chandran M, Candolfi M, Shah D, Mineharu Y, Yadav VN, Koschmann C, et al. Single vs. combination immunotherapeutic strategies for glioma. Expert Opinion on Biological Therapy. May 2017;**17**(5):543-554

[98] Hartmann J, Schussler-Lenz M, Bondanza A, Buchholz CJ. Clinical development of CAR T cells-challenges and opportunities in translating innovative treatment concepts. EMBO Molecular Medicine. Sep 2017;**9**(9):1183-1197

[99] Greco R, Oliveira G, Stanghellini MT, Vago L, Bondanza A, Peccatori J, et al. Improving the safety of cell therapy with the TK-suicide gene. Frontiers in Pharmacology. 2015;**6**:95

[100] Casucci M, Nicolis di Robilant B, Falcone L, Camisa B, Norelli M, Genovese P, et al. CD44v6-targeted T cells mediate potent antitumor effects against acute myeloid leukemia and multiple myeloma. Blood Nov 14, 2013;**122**(20):3461-3472

[101] Di Stasi A, Tey SK, Dotti G, Fujita Y, Kennedy-Nasser A, Martinez C, et al. Inducible apoptosis as a safety switch for adoptive cell therapy. The New England Journal of Medicine. Nov 3, 2011;**365**(18):1673-1683

[102] Strauss BE, Costanzi-Strauss E. pCLPG: A p53-driven retroviral system. Virology. Apr 10, 2004;**321**(2):165-172

[103] Bajgelman MC, Medrano RF, Carvalho AC, Strauss BE. AAVPG: A vigilant vector where transgene expression is induced by p53. Virology. Dec 2013;**447**(1-2):166-171

[104] Tamura RE, da Silva Soares RB, Costanzi-Strauss E, Strauss BE. Autoregulated expression of p53 from an adenoviral vector confers superior tumor inhibition in a model of prostate carcinoma gene therapy. Cancer Biology & Therapy. Dec 2016;**17**(12):1221-1230

[105] Strauss BE, Bajgelman MC, Costanzi-Strauss E. A novel gene transfer strategy that combines promoter and transgene activities for improved tumor cell inhibition. Cancer Gene Therapy. Dec 2005;**12**(12):935-946

[106] Tamura RE, Hunger A, Fernandes DC, Laurindo FR, Costanzi-Strauss E, Strauss BE. Induction of oxidants distinguishes susceptibility of prostate carcinoma cell lines to p53 gene transfer mediated by an improved adenoviral vector. Human Gene Therapy. Aug 2017;**28**(8):639-653

[107] Merkel CA, da Silva Soares RB, de Carvalho AC, Zanatta DB, Bajgelman MC, Fratini P, et al. Activation of endogenous p53 by combined p19Arf gene transfer and nutlin-3 drug treatment modalities in the murine cell lines B16 and C6. BMC Cancer. Jun 22, 2010;**10**:316

[108] Cui Y, Guo G. Immunomodulatory function of the tumor suppressor p53 in host immune response and the tumor microenvironment. International Journal of Molecular Sciences. Nov 19, 2016;**17**(11):e1942

[109] Medrano RFV, Hunger A, Mendonca SA, Barbuto JAM, Strauss BE. Immunomodulatory and antitumor effects of type I interferons and their application in cancer therapy. Oncotarget. Sep 19, 2017;**8**(41):71249-71284

[110] Merkel CA, Medrano RF, Barauna VG, Strauss BE. Combined p19Arf and interferon-beta gene transfer enhances cell death of B16 melanoma in vitro and in vivo. Cancer Gene Therapy. May 2013;**20**(5):317-325

[111] Hunger A, Medrano RF, Zanatta DB, Del Valle PR, Merkel CA, Salles TA, et al. Reestablishment of p53/Arf and interferon-beta pathways mediated by a novel adenoviral vector potentiates antiviral response and immunogenic cell death. Cell Death Discovery. 2017;**3**:17017

[112] Medrano RF, Catani JP, Ribeiro AH, Tomaz SL, Merkel CA, Costanzi-Strauss E, et al. Vaccination using melanoma cells treated with p19arf and interferon beta gene transfer in a mouse model: A novel combination for cancer immunotherapy. Cancer Immunology, Immunotherapy. Apr 2016;**65**(4):371-382

[113] Catani JP, Medrano RF, Hunger A, Del Valle P, Adjemian S, Zanatta DB, et al. Intratumoral immunization by p19Arf and interferon-beta gene transfer in a heterotopic mouse model of lung carcinoma. Translational Oncology. Dec 2016;**9**(6):565-574

[114] Medrano RFV, Hunger A, Catani JPP, Strauss BE. Uncovering the immunotherapeutic cycle initiated by p19Arf and interferon-beta gene transfer to cancer cells: An inducer of immunogenic cell death. Oncoimmunology. 2017;**6**(7):e1329072

[115] Hunger A, Medrano RF, Strauss BE. Harnessing combined p19Arf and interferon-beta gene transfer as an inducer of immunogenic cell death and mediator of cancer immunotherapy. Cell Death & Disease. May 11, 2017;**8**(5):e2784

[116] Strauss BE, Silva GRO, Vieira IDL, Cerqueira OLD, Valle PRD, Medrano RFV, et al. Perspectives for cancer immunotherapy mediated by p19Arf plus interferon-beta gene transfer. Clinics. 2018;**73**:e479s

[117] Dock G. The influence of complicating diseases upon leukaemia. The American Journal of the Medical Sciences. 1904;**127**:561-592

[118] Hoster HA, Zanes RP, Von Haam E. Studies in Hodgkin's syndrome; the association of viral hepatitis and Hodgkin's disease; a preliminary report. Cancer Research. Aug 1949;**9**(8):473-480

[119] Newman W, Southam CM. Virus treatment in advanced cancer: A pathological study of fifty-seven cases. Cancer. Jan 1954;**7**(1):106-118

[120] Kelly E, Russell SJ. History of oncolytic viruses: Genesis to genetic engineering. Molecular Therapy: The Journal of the American Society of Gene Therapy. Apr 2007;**15**(4): 651-659

[121] Martuza RL, Malick A, Markert JM, Ruffner KL, Coen DM. Experimental therapy of human glioma by means of a genetically engineered virus mutant. Science. May 1991;**252**(5007):854-856

[122] Moore AE. Viruses with oncolytic properties and their adaptation to tumors. Annals of the New York Academy of Sciences. Jul 1952;**54**(6):945-952

[123] Kauffman MG, Kelly TJ. Cell cycle regulation of thymidine kinase: Residues near the carboxyl terminus are essential for the specific degradation of the enzyme at mitosis. Molecular and Cellular Biology. May 1991;**11**(5):2538-2546

[124] Kelly EJ, Russell SJ. MicroRNAs and the regulation of vector tropism. Molecular Therapy: The Journal of the American Society of Gene Therapy. Mar 2009;**17**(3):409-416

[125] Verheije MH, Rottier PJ. Retargeting of viruses to generate oncolytic agents. Advances in Virology. 2012;**2012**:798526

[126] Rodriguez R, Schuur ER, Lim HY, Henderson GA, Simons JW, Henderson DR. Prostate attenuated replication competent adenovirus (ARCA) CN706: A selective cytotoxic for prostate-specific antigen-positive prostate cancer cells. Cancer Research. Jul 1997; **57**(13):2559-2563

[127] Tollefson AE, Scaria A, Hermiston TW, Ryerse JS, Wold LJ, Wold WS. The adenovirus death protein (E3-11.6K) is required at very late stages of infection for efficient cell lysis and release of adenovirus from infected cells. Journal of Virology. Apr 1996;**70**(4):2296-2306

[128] Tollefson AE, Ryerse JS, Scaria A, Hermiston TW, Wold WS. The E3-11.6-kDa adenovirus death protein (ADP) is required for efficient cell death: Characterization of cells infected with ADP mutants. Virology. Jun 1996;**220**(1):152-162

[129] Jhawar SR, Thandoni A, Bommareddy PK, Hassan S, Kohlhapp FJ, Goyal S, et al. Oncolytic viruses-natural and genetically engineered cancer immunotherapies. Frontiers in Oncology. 2017;**7**:202

[130] de Gruijl TD, Janssen AB, van Beusechem VW. Arming oncolytic viruses to leverage antitumor immunity. Expert Opinion on Biological Therapy. Jul 2015;**15**(7):959-971

[131] Frew SE, Sammut SM, Shore AF, Ramjist JK, Al-Bader S, Rezaie R, et al. Chinese health biotech and the billion-patient market. Nature Biotechnology. Jan 2008;**26**(1):37-53

[132] Liang M. Oncorine, the world first oncolytic virus medicine and its update in China. Current Cancer Drug Targets. 2018;**18**(2):171-176

[133] Wei D, Xu J, Liu XY, Chen ZN, Bian H. Fighting cancer with viruses: Oncolytic virus therapy in China. Human Gene Therapy. Feb 2018;**29**(2):151-159

[134] O'Shea CC, Soria C, Bagus B, McCormick F. Heat shock phenocopies E1B-55K late functions and selectively sensitizes refractory tumor cells to ONYX-015 oncolytic viral therapy. Cancer Cell. Jul 2005;**8**(1):61-74

[135] Galanis E, Okuno SH, Nascimento AG, Lewis BD, Lee RA, Oliveira AM, et al. Phase I-II trial of ONYX-015 in combination with MAP chemotherapy in patients with advanced sarcomas. Gene Therapy. Mar 2005;**12**(5):437-445

[136] Chiocca EA, Abbed KM, Tatter S, Louis DN, Hochberg FH, Barker F, et al. A phase I open-label, dose-escalation, multi-institutional trial of injection with an E1B-attenuated adenovirus, ONYX-015, into the peritumoral region of recurrent malignant gliomas, in the adjuvant setting. Molecular Therapy. Nov 2004;**10**(5):958-966

[137] Reid TR, Freeman S, Post L, McCormick F, Sze DY. Effects of Onyx-015 among metastatic colorectal cancer patients that have failed prior treatment with 5-FU/leucovorin. Cancer Gene Therapy. Aug 2005;**12**(8):673-681

[138] Makower D, Rozenblit A, Kaufman H, Edelman M, Lane ME, Zwiebel J, et al. Phase II clinical trial of intralesional administration of the oncolytic adenovirus ONYX-015 in patients with hepatobiliary tumors with correlative p53 studies. Clinical Cancer Research. Feb 2003;**9**(2):693-702

[139] Hu JC, Coffin RS, Davis CJ, Graham NJ, Groves N, Guest PJ, et al. A phase I study of OncoVEXGM-CSF, a second-generation oncolytic herpes simplex virus expressing granulocyte macrophage colony-stimulating factor. Clinical Cancer Research. Nov 2006;**12**(22):6737-6747

[140] Senzer NN, Kaufman HL, Amatruda T, Nemunaitis M, Reid T, Daniels G, et al. Phase II clinical trial of a granulocyte-macrophage colony-stimulating factor-encoding, second-generation oncolytic herpesvirus in patients with unresectable metastatic melanoma. Journal of Clinical Oncology. Dec 2009;**27**(34):5763-5771

[141] Andtbacka RH, Kaufman HL, Collichio F, Amatruda T, Senzer N, Chesney J, et al. Talimogene laherparepvec improves durable response rate in patients with advanced melanoma. Journal of Clinical Oncology. Sep 2015;**33**(25):2780-2788

[142] Wu AA, Drake V, Huang HS, Chiu S, Zheng L. Reprogramming the tumor microenvironment: Tumor-induced immunosuppressive factors paralyze T cells. Oncoimmunology. Jul 2015;**4**(7):e1016700

[143] Lim WA, June CH. The principles of engineering immune cells to treat Cancer. Cell. Feb 9, 2017;**168**(4):724-740

[144] D'Aloia MM, Zizzari IG, Sacchetti B, Pierelli L, Alimandi M. CAR-T cells: The long and winding road to solid tumors. Cell Death & Disease. Feb 2018;**9**(3):282

[145] Prasad V. Immunotherapy: Tisagenlecleucel—The first approved CAR-T-cell therapy: Implications for payers and policy makers. Nature Reviews. Clinical Oncology. Jan 2018;**15**(1):11-12

[146] Alissa Poh. FDA approves second CAR T-cell therapy. Cancer Discovery. Jan 2018; **8**(1):5-6

[147] Badieyan ZS, Hoseini SS. Adverse effects associated with clinical applications of CAR engineered T cells. Archivum Immunologiae et Therapiae Experimentalis (Warsz). Aug 2018;**66**(4):283-288

[148] Smith TT, Stephan SB, Moffett HF, McKnight LE, Ji W, Reiman D, et al. In situ programming of leukaemia-specific T cells using synthetic DNA nanocarriers. Nature Nanotechnology. Aug 2017;**12**(8):813-820

[149] Chen DS, Mellman I. Oncology meets immunology: The cancer-immunity cycle. Immunity. Jul 25, 2013;**39**(1):1-10

Chapter 6

AAV-Mediated Gene Therapy for *CRB1*-Hereditary Retinopathies

Celso Henrique Alves and Jan Wijnholds

Additional information is available at the end of the chapter

http://dx.doi.org/10.5772/intechopen.79308

Abstract

Variations in the Crumbs homolog-1 (*CRB1*) gene lead to autosomal recessive retinal dystrophies such as early-onset retinitis pigmentosa (RP) and Leber congenital amaurosis (LCA). No treatment is yet available for these patients. Adeno-associated virus (AAV) mediated gene therapy for hereditary retinal diseases holds great promise proven by the large number of active clinical trials. We here summarized the knowledge about the localization and function of CRB1 in the retina and the main pathological features resulting from loss of CRB1 function in humans and in rodents. This know-how is being applied to design and develop AAV gene therapy vectors for the treatment of *CRB1*-Hereditary retinopathies. Knowing which cell types express the CRB proteins, the possible redundancy of function between CRB1 and CRB2, and the AAV tropism in the human retina, will allow us to rationalize about the AAV capsid, promoter and route of administration that should be used in the AAV vector in order to efficiently and specifically deliver *CRB1* or *CRB2* into the human retina.

Keywords: crumbs homolog-1 (CRB1), retinitis pigmentosa, Leber congenital amaurosis, gene therapy, adeno-associated virus (AAV)

1. Introduction

A new generation of medicines emerged in 2012 with the first ever European market authorization of Glybera (alipogene tiparvovec), an adeno-associated virus (AAV) gene therapy medicine for the treatment of a rare inherited autosomal recessive lipid disorder, lipoprotein lipase deficiency. Five years later the company did not seek for renewal of the marketing authorization for Glybera due to patient's lack of demand [1]. Despite the marketing failure

Targeted disease	AAV serotype	Promoter	Gene	Delivery route	Volume injected	Dosage	ClinicalTrials.gov Identifier	Ref.
LCA	AAV4	RPE65	*hRPE65*	Subretinal	400 or 800 μL	1.22×10^{10} vg 4.8×10^{10} vg	NCT01496040	[17]
	AAV2	CBA	*hRPE65*	Subretinal	450 μL	1.8×10^{11} vg 6×10^{11} vg	NCT00749957	[18, 19]
	AAV2	hRPE65	*hRPE65*	Subretinal	up to 1 mL	up to 3×10^{12} vg	NCT00643747	[4, 20]
	AAV2	CB^{SB}	*hRPE65*	Subretinal	150–300 μL	8.94×10^{9} 3.58×10^{10} vg	NCT00481546	[21]
	AAV2	CBA	*hRPE65v2*	Subretinal	150 μL	1.5×10^{10} vg 4.8×10^{10} vg 1.5×10^{11} vg	NCT00999609	[22]
Choroideremia	AAV2	CBA	*REP1*	Subretinal	60–100 μL	10^{10}–10^{11} vg	NCT01461213 NCT02407678 NCT02077361	[5]
	AAV2	NR	*hCHM*	Subretinal	NR	NR	NCT02341807	NR
RP (*RLBP1*)	AAV8	sRLBP1 CPK850	*hRLBP1*	Subretinal	NR	NR	NCT03374657	[23]
RP (*PDE6B*)	AAV5	RK	*hPDE6B*	Subretinal	NR	NR	NCT03328130	[24]
RP (*MERTK*)	AAV2	VMD2	*hMERTK*	Subretinal	NR	NR	NCT01482195	[25]
X-linked RP	NR	NR	*RPGR*	Subretinal	NR	NR	NCT03116113	NR
	AAV2tYF	GRK1	*RPGR*	Subretinal	NR	NR	NCT03316560	[26, 27]
Achromatopsia	AAV8	NRx	*hCNGA3*	Subretinal	NR	1×10^{10} vg 5×10^{10} vg 1×10^{11} vg	NCT02610582	NR
	AAV8	hCAR	*CNGB3*	Subretinal	NR	NR	NCT03001310	NR
	AAV2tYF	PR1.7	*CNGA3*	Subretinal	NR	NR	NCT02935517	[28]
	AAV2tYF	PR1.7	*CNGB3*	Subretinal	NR	NR	NCT02599922	[29]
X-linked retinoschisis	AAV8	scRS/IRBP	*shRS*	Intravitreal	NR	NR	NCT02317887	[30, 31]
	AAV2tYF	CB	*hRS1*	Intravitreal	NR	NR	NCT02416622	[32]
Leber hereditary optic neuropathy (LHON)	scAAV2 (Y444,500,730F)	CMV/CBA	*P1ND4v2*	Intravitreal	200 μL	5.00×10^{9} vg 2.46×10^{10} vg 1.0×10^{11} vg	NCT02161380	[8, 33]
	AAV2	CMV	*ND4*	Intravitreal	90 μL	3×10^{10} vg $9 \times x10^{10}$ vg 1.8×10^{11} vg	NCT02064569 NCT02652767 NCT02652780 NCT03293524	[34, 35]

Targeted disease	AAV serotype	Promoter	Gene	Delivery route	Volume injected	Dosage	ClinicalTrials. gov Identifier	Ref.
Age-Related Macular Degeneration (AMD)	AAV2	CMV	*sFLT01*	Intravitreal	100 μL	2×10^8 vg 2×10^9 vg 6×10^9 vg 2×10^{10} vg	NCT01024998	[36]
	AAV8	NR	*soluble anti-VEGF*	Subretinal	NR	3×10^9 vg 1×10^{10} vg 6×10^{10} vg	NCT03066258	NR

CBA: chicken β-actin promoter (CBA); CB^{SB}: Hybrid modified short cytomegalovirus (CMV) enhancer and chicken β-actin promoter (CBA); GRK1: G protein-coupled receptor kinase; hCAR: human cone arrestin; NR: not reported; PR1.7: 1.7-kb L-opsin promoter; REF: References; RK: Rhodopsin kinase; scRS/IRBP: Retinoschisin/interphotoreceptor retinoid binding protein; VMD2: Vitelliform macular dystrophy-2.

Table 1. Summary of the clinical trials for retinopathies using AAV as delivery system registered on ClinicalTrials.gov database.

of Glybera, the use of AAV gene therapy in the eye is very attractive since the marketing prospects look better for the small amounts of AAV medicine to be transferred into the retinal tissue or retinal pigment epithelium. The eye is well accessible for surgery and allows direct observation, *in vivo*, of the retinal tissue in microscopic detail. Moreover, the eye is considered an immune-privileged tissue. Therefore, the risks of an immune response against the virus and/or the transgene itself are reduced. The local application in the "compartmentalized" eye of low amounts of AAV drug will minimize side effects expected if systemically applied at high doses [2]. But most importantly, potential drug efficacy for retinal orphan diseases can be efficiently proven thanks to a plethora of non-invasive retinal investigation techniques.

At the end of 2017, Luxturna (voretigene neparvovec-rzyl) became the first FDA-approved AAV gene therapy medicine for patients with hereditary retinal disease caused by biallelic *RPE65* gene mutations [3, 4]. The market approvals of the first gene therapy medicines in Europa and in the USA paved the road to similar programs, reflected on the large number of clinical trials registered on the ClinicalTrials.gov website using AAVs as a delivery strategy to treat hereditary retinal diseases such as choroideremia (*CHM* or *REP-1*) [5], achromatopsia (*CNGA3*) [6], wet age-related macular degeneration (AMD) (*VEGFR1/FLT* and a gene encoding soluble anti-VEGF protein) [7], Leber hereditary optic neuropathy (LHON) (*ND4*) [8], autosomal recessive retinitis pigmentosa (arRP) (*MERTK*) [9], X-linked RP (*RPGR*) [10], RP (*PDE6B*) [11] and (*RLBP1*) [12] and X-linked Retinoschisis (*RS1*) [13, 14] (**Table 1**). Developing an AAV gene therapy to treat patients with mutations in the Crumbs homolog-1 (*CRB1*) gene was particularly challenging due to its large cDNA (4.2 kb) which approached the packaging limit of the AAV genome (~4.7–4.9 kb). Thus, to build an AAV vector that allowed efficient packaging of the human *CRB1* cDNA, the use of a short promoter (<350 bp) and a short synthetic polyadenylation sequence was required to efficiently express the CRB1 protein *in vivo*. Codon optimization of the *CRB1* cDNA was used to achieve sufficient levels of expression [15]. A second strategy that implied the replacement of CRB1 by its structural and functional family member CRB2 was used to overcome the size limitation and potential toxicity due to expression of CRB1. *CRB2* cDNA was only

3.85 kb in size and gave more flexibility to design the AAV gene therapy vector in terms of promoter sequence size, polyadenylation sequence and other optimized sequences that stabilized the transcript [16].

2. *CRB1*-Hereditary retinopathies

More than 240 different mutations in the *CRB1* gene have been described so far (http://www.LOVD.nl/CRB1). These gene variations are associated with a wide variety of retinal dystrophies, including autosomal recessive retinitis pigmentosa (RP), Leber congenital amaurosis (LCA), cone-rod dystrophy, isolated macular dystrophy and foveal retinoschisis [37]. Furthermore, mutations in *CRB1* are responsible for 7–17% of all the LCA cases and for approximately 3–9% of all cases of RP [38, 39]. Retinitis pigmentosa type 12 (RP12) due to mutations in the *CRB1* gene was initially characterized by RP with preservation of para-arteriolar retinal pigment epithelium (PPRPE), progressive visual field loss starting from the first decades of life, and early macular involvement. Later on it became clear that RP12 commonly presents early-onset retinitis pigmentosa, hyperopia and optic disc drusen, with or without PPRPE [37, 40, 41]. Leber congenital amaurosis type 8, due to mutation in the *CRB1* gene (LCA8), is a severe form of retinal dystrophy characterized by roving eye movements or nystagmus, nonrecordable or severely reduced cone and rod electroretinography amplitudes and severe loss of vision within the first years of life. Retinas of LCA8 patients with *CRB1* mutations are about 1.5 times thicker than normal retinas, while retinas of patients with LCA due to mutations in other genes such as *RPE65* or *GUCY2D* are thinner [42]. In addition, LCA8 retinas showed abnormal retinal architecture suggesting that loss of CRB1 function might interrupt the naturally occurring process of proliferation, apoptosis and cell migration during retinal development [42–44].

No treatment is yet available for *CRB1*-associated retinal dystrophies. We achieved proof-of-concept for retinal *CRB1* gene therapy, using an AAV9-CMV-*hCRB2* vector in two mouse models. A first model lacked CRB1 and had reduced levels of CRB2 in Müller glial cells and photoreceptors, and a second model lacked CRB2 from Müller glial cells and photoreceptors [16]. These two pre-clinical studies opened the perspective for therapeutic trials for human *CRB1*-associated dystrophies.

Intriguingly, there is no clear genotype–phenotype correlation for *CRB1* mutations [45]. This fact associated with the large spectrum of retinal dystrophies observed in patients with mutations in the *CRB1* gene [37], reinforced the need to study in detail the clinical features and natural disease progression of *CRB1*-associated retinal dystrophies before moving towards a clinical trial. This knowledge is required to establish patient eligibility criteria and clinical outcomes for the forthcoming clinical trial.

2.1. The *CRB1*-complex in the retina

In the developing mouse retina, the retinal neuroepithelium is composed of multipotent retinal progenitor cells that differentiate in a time-dependent manner, giving rise to six major types of neuronal and one type of glial cells. The first cell type to be generated from the progenitors are the ganglion cells, followed in overlapping sequential phases by horizontal cells, cone photoreceptors, amacrine cells, rod photoreceptors, bipolar cells and the Müller glial cells. The seven retinal cell types organize or "laminate" in three orderly distinct nuclear layers divided by two plexiform layers [46]. The CRB complex plays a crucial role during retinogenesis by the establishment of polarity, adhesion, retinal lamination and restricting proliferation and apoptosis of progenitors and the number of late born cells such as rod photoreceptors, bipolar cells, late-born amacrine cells and Müller glial cells [47–52].

The CRB family in mammals consists of three members CRB1, CRB2 and CRB3. Both the CRB1 and CRB2 have a large extracellular domain with epidermal growth factor-like and laminin-A globular domains, a single transmembrane domain and a short intracellular C-terminal domain. The C-terminal domain of 37 amino acids has a single FERM-protein-binding motif juxtaposed to the transmembrane domain and a single C-terminal PDZ protein-binding motif [53–55]. While CRB3, the third family member, contains the transmembrane and C-terminal domain but is very short in length since it lacks the large extracellular domain. The C-terminal PDZ motifs of CRB proteins bind to the PDZ domain of PALS1 (also called MPP5). PALS1 binds via its N-terminal L27 domain to the L27 domain of the multiple PDZ proteins PATJ and MUPP1 [56]. The multi-adapter protein PALS1 recruits MPP3 and MPP4 to the subapical protein complex at the so called subapical region adjacent to adherens junctions at the outer limiting membrane [57, 58]. Loss of the CRB1, CRB2, PALS1, or MPP3 but not MPP4 resulted in disruption of adhesion between photoreceptors and Müller glial cells. In summary, the core of the retinal CRB-complex is composed of CRB1, CRB2, PALS1, PATJ, MUPP1, and MPP3 [52, 59].

In the embryonic mouse retina, CRB1, CRB2, PALS1, PATJ and MUPP1 are expressed at the subapical region adjacent to the adherens junctions of the retinal progenitor cells [49]. In the adult mouse retina, CRB2 is present at the subapical region in photoreceptors and Müller glial cells. The mouse *Crb1* gene transcript is expressed in photoreceptors and Müller glial cells but expression of the CRB1 protein is limited to the subapical region of Müller glial cells [60, 61]. CRB3 has a broader expression pattern being located at the subapical region in both photoreceptors and Müller glial cells [52, 60], at the photoreceptor inner segments and photoreceptor synaptic terminals and at sub-populations of amacrine and bipolar cells in the inner plexiform layer [62]. The expression patterns of CRB1 and CRB2 observed in the mouse retina do in part match with the ones observed in the human retina. In the first trimester human fetal retina, CRB2 but not CRB1 is expressed at the subapical region. While in the second trimester CRB1, CRB2 and PALS1 localize at the subapical region. A similar expression pattern is observed in early (differentiation day 28) versus late (differentiation day 160) human induced pluripotent stem cells (iPSCs)-derived retinas [63]. Immunoelectron microscopic protein localization studies performed on adult human retinas, collected at two to 3 days post-mortem, showed CRB1 and CRB2 localization at the subapical region of Müller glial cells as found in the mouse retina. Human CRB1 localized also at the subapical region in photoreceptor cells, whereas human CRB2 localized at vesicles in the photoreceptor inner segments some distance away from the subapical region [52, 60] (**Figure 1**).

Interestingly, the overexpression of human CRB2 protein specifically in mouse photoreceptors that lacked endogenous mouse CRB2 in photoreceptors and Müller glial cells, caused aberrant localization of human CRB2 predominantly at vesicles in photoreceptor inner segments

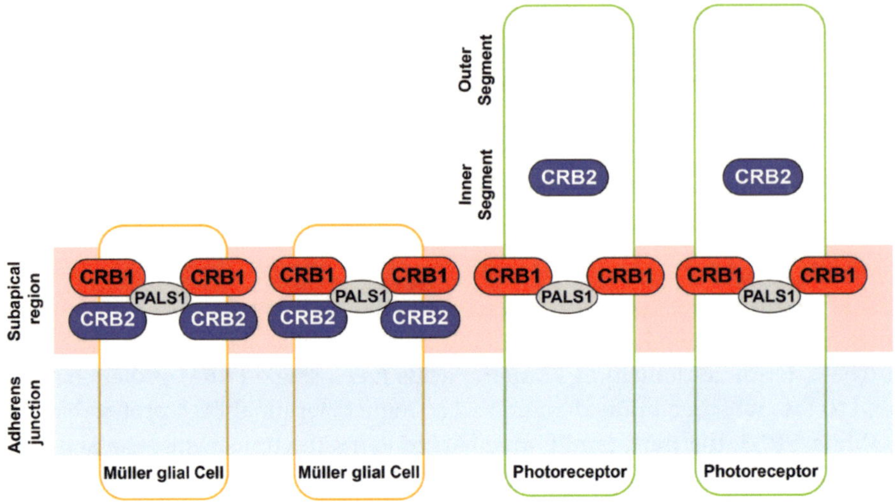

Figure 1. Model depicting the localization of CRB1 and CRB2 proteins in the human retina at 2 days post-mortem. CRB proteins are present at the subapical region above the adherens junctions between Müller glial cells, between photoreceptor and Müller glial cells and between photoreceptor cells. CRB1 is located in both Müller glial cells and cone and rod photoreceptor cells at the subapical region. CRB2 is located in Müller glial cells at the subapical region, and in photoreceptors at vesicles in the inner segments at a distance from the subapical region.

at a distance from the subapical region. However, when expressed in both photoreceptors and Müller glial cells, human CRB2 localization was restricted to the subapical region, which suggested that expression of CRB2 in both cells types might be required for proper protein localization and function [16].

2.2. Animal models for *CRB1*-retinopathies

Animal models able to recapitulate features of the *CRB1*-retinopathies are of value to understand the molecular mechanism behind retinopathies and to test new AAV gene therapy vectors. Over the recent years several rodent models were described in the literature. The retinal phenotypes observed in these animals mimic the wide spectrum of clinical features as described in *CRB1*-patients, including early and late onset RP, LCA and telangiectasia [44, 49, 50, 52, 64–67]. The onset and severity of the phenotype observed in these animal models seem closely associated with the total levels of the CRB proteins in the different cell compartments. The available models can be grouped into three major categories:

a. late onset-RP: homozygous knockout *Crb1* [52], hemizygous knockin $Crb1^{C249W/-}$ [67] and homozygous naturally occurring mutant $Crb1^{rd8}$ [66] mice showed, at foci, loss of integrity of the outer limiting membrane, with protrusions of rows of photoreceptor nuclei into the inner- and outer segments layer and ingression of photoreceptor nuclei into the photoreceptor synaptic layer. Microglial cell infiltration and upregulation of glial fibrillary acidic protein (GFAP) were observed at the foci of photoreceptor dysplasia. Conditional ablation of *Crb2* specifically in Müller glial cells resulted in disruptions at the outer limiting membrane and ectopic photoreceptor nuclei in the inner- and outer segment layer [50]. The morphological abnormalities observed in all these models do not lead to a decrease in electrical retinal function.

b. early onset-RP: ablation of *Crb2* from retinal progenitor cells, and consequent loss of CRB2 in cone and rod photoreceptors and Müller glial cells [47, 49] or ablation of *Crb2* specifically in immature photoreceptors [50] leads to disruptions at the outer limiting membrane during late-stage embryonic development resulting in abnormalities in retinal lamination, severe retinal degeneration and early loss of retinal function. More recently, a naturally occurring substrain of Brown Norway rats (BN-J) was described as a model for retinal telangiectasia due to homozygous variations in the *Crb1* gene. Interestingly the retinal phenotype observed in this *Crb1* rat strain differs from the phenotype observed in the *Crb1* knockout mice. The *Crb1* rat displays retinal dysplasia at early postnatal days, leading to early-onset disruption of photoreceptor synapses and subsequent loss of retinal function at 1 month of age and near to complete photoreceptor cell death at 6 months of age [64].

c. LCA: mouse retinas with loss of CRB1 and CRB2 proteins from retinal progenitor cells showed lack of a proper retinal lamination with loss of a photoreceptor synaptic layer, intermingling of photoreceptor nuclei with the nuclei of inner nuclear layer cells, and early loss of retinal function [44].

The lack of a genotype–phenotype correlation in humans might correlate with the different retinal phenotypes as observed in mice with lowered levels of CRB1 and/or CRB2 in retinal progenitors, photoreceptors and Müller glial cells. Cumulative data suggest that not only the levels of CRB1 are important for the pathogenesis observed in humans but also the total levels of CRB1 and CRB2 proteins. Or that the levels of functional CRB2 variants in retinal progenitors, photoreceptors or Müller glial cells might play a role in determining the severity of the retinal dystrophy caused by mutations in the *CRB1* gene.

3. Adeno-associated virus (AAV) biology

Adeno-associated virus belongs to the parvovirus family, but is placed in the genus Dependovirus since it is dependent on co-infection with other viruses, mainly adenoviruses, in order to replicate. AAV is a small, non-enveloped single-stranded DNA virus. The genome of the AAV is approximately 4.7 kb and has three open reading frames to express the *rep* (Replication), *cap* (Capsid) and assembly activating protein (*aap*) (Assembly) genes, flanked by two 145 nucleotide-long inverted terminal repeats (ITRs). The ITRs self-assemble into hairpin structures required for genome replication, integration and encapsidation. The *rep* gene encodes four proteins (Rep78, Rep68, Rep52 and Rep40), which are required for viral genome replication and packaging. While *cap* gene transcripts gives rise to the viral capsid proteins, virion protein 1 (VP1), VP2 and VP3, with molecular weights of 87, 72 and 62 kDa, respectively. These capsid proteins assemble into an icosahedral symmetry protein shell of 60 subunits, in a molar ratio of 1:1:10 (VP1:VP2:VP3). The *aap* gene encodes the assembly-activating protein (AAP) that is thought to have a scaffolding function for capsid assembly [68]. Wild-type AAV integrates into the human host genome at a specific site, AAVS1 on chromosome 19.

In gene therapy a recombinant AAV (rAAV) and not the wild-type AAV are used. In rAAV the viral genome required for viral replication, the rep and *cap* genes, and the element required for site-specific integration are deleted. A sequence containing a promoter, a 5′-untranslated region, the cDNA of a transgene of interest, and a 3′-untranslated region containing a polyadenylation site are then inserted in between the AAV vector containing the two ITRs. To produce AAV particles from the AAV gene therapy plasmid in a human cell line, the *rep* and *cap* genes are supplied in trans on a helper plasmid along with helper genes from adenovirus (*E4*, *E2a* and *VA*) necessary for replication.

The major advantages of the use of rAAVs are the safety profile, low immunogenicity, lack of toxicity and the property that the rAAV genomes do not integrate into the host genome. The rAAV capsid enters the cells by receptor-mediated endocytosis, the rAAV genomes are processed into nuclear episomal structures and are maintained extrachromosomally. Dependent on the gene therapy vector used, and the life span of the targeted cell, the rAAV genomes can express a transgene for more than 10 years. AAV vectors also have the ability to transduce non-dividing cells, including non-dividing retinal neurons like photoreceptors. One major disadvantage of the rAAV technology is the size limitation of the total DNA that can be efficiently packaged in the AAV vector (4.7–4.9 kb) which makes it difficult to design AAV-mediated gene therapy for larger genes (≥ 4 kb). The development of dual and triple AAV vectors with a maximum transfer capacity of around 9 and 14 kb, respectively, might in the future overcome in part this limitation [69].

The generation of a gene therapy vector able to deliver CRB1 is particularly challenging due to its large size of cDNA (4.2 kb). To assemble the gene therapy vector, the 4.2 kb *CRB1 cDNA* and the two ITR sequences (0.29 kb) need to be added which make up to 4.49 kb. Therefore, only 0.2–0.41 kb space is left for the promoter and polyadenylation sequences. Although challenging it was shown that it is possible to efficiently package human *CRB1 cDNA* in AAV vectors and to express CRB1 protein *in vivo* [15, 16]. Another strategy to overcome the size limitation is to use the 3.85 kb *CRB2 cDNA* as replacement [16].

3.1. Gene delivery in the retina using AAVs

The eye offers a set of unique features for the application of gene therapy vectors. The eye is a small, compartmentalized, immunoprivileged, paired organ and easily accessible using minimally invasive techniques. There are also high resolution functional and structural diagnostics, such as, optical coherence tomography, scanning laser ophthalmoscopy and electroretinography, as well as psychophysical tests such as microperimetry, kinetic perimetry, visual acuity testing, and multi-luminance mobility test (MLMT) in the ophthalmology field that allow to examine the eye/retina structure and to test as well retinal function and vision. Gene therapy vectors for retinal disease can be delivered mainly by two routes: subretinally into the "subretinal space" between the neural retina and the RPE, or intravitreally, into the vitreous body, both approaches are described below. The administration route is an important parameter to take into consideration in the testing of gene therapy vectors, together with the selection of the AAV capsid and promoter since all these parameters have effects on the tropism of the vectors.

3.2. Route of delivery

3.2.1. Subretinal injection

In pre-clinical studies performed in rodents *ab externo* subretinal injections are commonly performed [16, 70]. This method uses a small needle (34 gauge) to penetrate (*ab externo*) the sclera at the limbus and under direct observation the needle can be guided through the retina to create a subretinal space between the retinal pigment epithelium and the outer limiting membrane. Normally, a volume of 1 μL is injected to form an injection fluid bleb that transiently detaches a large portion of neural retina from the RPE in one single injection. Incorrect surgery might cause cataract due to damage to the lens. It is also common to have a large volume of backflow of injected AAV particles when the injection needle is retracted.

Subretinal injections in human can be performed using the "single-step" or the "two-step" approach [71]. With the "single-step" approach the fluid, containing the gene therapy vector, is directly delivered into the subretinal space without previous retinal detachment [22].

The "two-step" approach consists of first the generation of a bleb in the subretinal space by injection of a balanced salt solution (BSS), followed by injection of the therapeutic agent using a controlled flow rate [4, 5, 72]. The second approach offers several advantages like the possibility to better assess the direction of bleb spread as well as to minimize vector loss by misguided injection [71]. The subretinal surgery and injection is a specialized technique and can in principle be executed by surgeons operating an ophthalmic surgery robot to obtain most reproducible results. According to information collected from the different clinical trials registered in the *Clinicaltrials.gov* database, a volume ranging from 60 to 1000 μL can be injected via this route (**Table 1**).

Subretinal injections seem the logical choice when RPE or photoreceptors are the target cells, since these cells will be in direct contact with the fluid containing the AAV particles. However, degenerating retinas at an advanced stage are often quite thin, with disruptions at the outer limiting membrane, loss of inner/outer segments and/or photoreceptor cells, neovascularization and infiltration of microglial cells. All these features might lead to a reduction in the potential subretinal space between the neural retina and the RPE, or to leaking of the AAV vector to the choroid vasculature system and influence the AAV tropism. The retinal detachment caused during the subretinal injection might potentially also either aggravate or alleviate the processes of retinal degeneration.

3.2.2. Intravitreal injection

Intravitreal injection implies direct delivery into the space in the back of the eye called the vitreous cavity, which is filled with a jelly-like fluid called the vitreous humor gel. Intravitreal injections are generally limited to volumes of up to 2 μL in mice [15, 16, 73], while in rats the volumes are limited to 3–5 μL [74]. The main surgical complications observed are cataract formation due to lens-induced damage and retinal perforation [75].

In humans intravitreal injections are generally performed under local anesthesia [71], by inserting a 30 gauge needle through the sclera at the pars plana region, 3.5–4 mm posterior to the limbus between vertical and horizontal muscles with limited reflux [71, 73]. In clinical trials volumes between 90 and 200 μL have been injected via this route (**Table 1**).

Intravitreal administration of AAV gene therapy might look tempting since it is an easier procedure with less potential surgical complications compared to the subretinal injection, especially when treating thinned degenerative retinas. However, administration of AAV intravitreally has its own caveats namely the difficulty of AAV capsids to cross the thick inner limiting membrane in the human retina and the current lack of AAV serotypes capable of transducing efficiently the human photoreceptors or RPE cells. Another obstacle is the potential AAV transduction and subsequent expression in other eye tissues, as for example, the ciliary body especially when using a ubiquitous promoter.

Pre-clinical studies in mice and rats showed that Müller glial cells can efficiently be infected after intravitreal administration of AAV2/6 or AAV2/shH10^{Y445F} [15, 76], therefore these AAV capsids might be used to deliver CRB1 or CRB2 into Müller cells. AAV serotype shH10^{Y445F} is however known to transduce efficiently the ciliary body epithelium when applied intravitreally [16].

3.3. AAV capsids and cell type specific promoters

The existence of 11 natural AAV serotypes and derivatives that differ in their tropism, and the different types of cells they infect, makes AAV a very useful system to infect the various cell types of the retina. The cell specificity of the AAV vector can be further increased by using cell type specific promoters, for example RPE65 or VMD2 to drive expression in retinal pigment epithelium. Or by using e.g. the rhodopsin (RH), G protein-coupled receptor kinase 1 (GRK1), 1.7-kb L-opsin promoter (PR1.7) or cone arrestin (hCAR) promoter to drive expression in rod and/or cone photoreceptors. Or using e.g. the RLBP1, GFAP or NR2E1 promoter to drive expression in Müller cells [17, 23, 24, 28].

Several pre-clinical studies showed the tropism and/or potency of the different capsids and promoter (cell specific or ubiquitous) in infecting retinal cell types such as RPE, photoreceptors and Müller glial cells. However, AAV tropism might differ *in vivo* between rodent species, dogs, non-human primates and human. AAV tropism is dependent of the route of administration, the stage of retinal development and severity of retinal dystrophy. Therefore, is quite difficult to extrapolate the data from pre-clinical studies performed in rodents directly to the human *in vivo* setting. To obtain evidence-based data for clinical gene therapy studies, researchers optimize culture protocols for human retinal organotypic cultures [77–79] or human iPSC-derived retinas to study the AAV tropism [80]. Recently, the capacity of different AAV serotypes to infect and express in human retinal cells was studied in organotypic cultures. This study suggested that serotypes AAV4, AAV5 and AAV6 were particularly efficient at transducing photoreceptor cells, whereas serotype AAV8 displayed consistently low transduction of these cells [79, 81]. Actually several AAV serotypes and ubiquitous promoters or cell specific promoters are being used in clinical trials (**Table 1**), the results from these studies will provide us with important clues about the best promoters and capsids to use in the human retina.

In order to deliver *CRB1* or *CRB2* into rod and cone photoreceptor and Müller glial cells in the human retina an AAV capsid able to infect all the three cell types needs to be used in combination with a promoter active in the same cells. Studies performed in mice suggested that a combination of AAV9 and a CMV promoter might be a possibility but further studies are required to test its suitability for human retinal cells [16]. Subretinal injection of expression vectors packaged into serotypes AAV5 or AAV9 infect photoreceptors *in vivo* in macaques [82, 83]. Tropism studies in human retinal explants reported that AAV5 would be more efficacious than AAV9 [84]. Another strategy would be the use of one vector to deliver *CRB1* or *CRB2* specifically in Müller glial cells and a second vector to deliver specifically in photoreceptors. Besides regulatory and financial issues, the main technical issues here resides with the lack of a short promoter (≤ 300 bp) specific for Müller cells, and the lack of an AAV serotype that in human retina efficiently infects Müller glial cells upon intravitreal or subretinal injection.

4. Conclusion

In recent years the scientific progress in the field of gene therapy for inherited retinal dystrophies culminated in the first ever approved AAV gene therapy medicine to treat LCA patients carrying mutations in the *RPE65* gene. The number of engineered AAV capsid variants and new promoters to drive expression in the different retinal cell types is raising at great speed allowing the design of more specific and more efficient viral vectors. Likewise, the number of clinical trials using AAV gene therapy is increasing at a similar rhythm, the data collected from these studies will be very useful for the development of similar therapies. Pre-clinical studies performed in mice demonstrated that AAV-mediated *CRB2* gene augmentation therapy might be a promising medicine to prevent progression of retinitis pigmentosa in patients with mutations in the *CRB1* gene. In mice at mid-stage retinal disease *CRB2* gene augmentation therapy successfully improved retinal morphology with preservation of photoreceptor cells and retinal function, therefore providing good perspectives for the forthcoming clinical trial in patients with RP due to mutations in *CRB1*.

Acknowledgements

This work was supported by ZonMw project nr 43200004; FFB project nr TA-GT-0715-0665-LUMC.

Conflict of interest

The LUMC is the holder of patent application PCT/NL2014/050549, which describes the potential clinical use of CRB2; JW is listed as inventor on this patent, and JW is an employee of the LUMC.

Author details

Celso Henrique Alves[1] and Jan Wijnholds[1,2*]

*Address all correspondence to: j.wijnholds@lumc.nl

1 Department of Ophthalmology, Leiden University Medical Center (LUMC), Leiden, The Netherlands

2 Netherlands Institute for Neuroscience, Royal Netherlands Academy of Arts and Sciences (KNAW), Amsterdam, The Netherlands

References

[1] Glybera. Glybera, INN - alipogene tiparvovec [Internet]. 2015. Available from: http://www.ema.europa.eu/docs/en_GB/document_library/EPAR_-_Summary_for_the_public/human/002145/WC500135474.pdf [Accessed: 2018-03-21]

[2] Hinderer C, Katz N, Buza EL, Dyer C, Goode T, Bell P, et al. Severe toxicity in nonhuman primates and piglets following high-dose intravenous administration of an AAV vector expressing human SMN. Human Gene Therapy. 2018;**29**(3):285-298

[3] LUXTURNATM. FDA Approves Spark Therapeutics' LUXTURNATM (voretigene neparvovec-rzyl), a One-time Gene Therapy for Patients with Confirmed Biallelic RPE65 Mutation-associated Retinal Dystrophy | Spark Therapeutics Inc. – IR Site [Internet]. 2018. Available from: http://ir.sparktx.com/news-releases/news-release-details/fda-approves-spark-therapeutics-luxturnatm-voretigene-neparvovec [Accessed: 2018-03-21]

[4] Bainbridge JW, Smith AJ, Barker SS, Robbie S, Henderson R, Balaggan K, et al. Effect of gene therapy on visual function in Leber's congenital Amaurosis. The New England Journal of Medicine. 2008;**358**(21):2231-2239

[5] MacLaren RE, Groppe M, Barnard AR, Cottriall CL, Tolmachova T, Seymour L, et al. Retinal gene therapy in patients with choroideremia: Initial findings from a phase 1/2 clinical trial. Lancet. 2014;**383**(9923):1129-1137

[6] Michalakis S, Mühlfriedel R, Tanimoto N, Krishnamoorthy V, Koch S, Fischer MD, et al. Restoration of cone vision in the CNGA3$^{-/-}$ mouse model of congenital complete lack of cone photoreceptor function. Molecular Therapy. 2010;**18**(12):2057-2063

[7] Sanofi-Genzyme. Safety and Tolerability Study of AAV2- sFLT01 in Patients With Neovascular Age-Related Macular Degeneration (AMD). [Internet]. 2016. Available from: http://clinicaltrials.gov/ct2/show/NCT01024998 [Accessed: 2018-03-21]

[8] Feuer WJ, Schiffman JC, Davis JL, Porciatti V, Gonzalez P, Koilkonda RD, et al. Gene therapy for Leber hereditary optic neuropathy: Initial results. Ophthalmology. 2016; **123**(3):558-570

[9] Ghazi NG, Abboud EB, Nowilaty SR, Alkuraya H, Alhommadi A, Cai H, et al. Treatment of retinitis pigmentosa due to MERTK mutations by ocular subretinal injection of adeno-associated virus gene vector: Results of a phase I trial. Human Genetics. 2016; **135**(3):327-343

[10] Beltran WA, Cideciyan AV, Boye SE, Ye GJ, Iwabe S, Dufour VL, et al. Optimization of retinal gene therapy for X-linked retinitis Pigmentosa due to RPGR mutations. Molecular Therapy. 2017;**25**(8):1866-1880

[11] Pang JJ, Boye SL, Kumar A, Dinculescu A, Deng W, Li J, et al. AAV-mediated gene therapy for retinal degeneration in the rd10 mouse containing a recessive PDEβ mutation. Investigative Ophthalmology and Visual Science. 2008;**49**(10):4278-4283

[12] Choi VW, Bigelow CE, McGee TL, Gujar AN, Li H, Hanks SM, et al. AAV-mediated RLBP1 gene therapy improves the rate of dark adaptation in Rlbp1 knockout mice. Molecular Therapy - Methods & Clinical Development. 2015;**2**:15022

[13] Ou J, Vijayasarathy C, Ziccardi L, Chen S, Zeng Y, Marangoni D, et al. Synaptic pathology and therapeutic repair in adult retinoschisis mouse by AAV-RS1 transfer. The Journal of Clinical Investigation. 2015;**125**(7):2891-2903

[14] Janssen A, Min SH, Molday LL, Tanimoto N, Seeliger MW, Hauswirth WW, et al. Effect of late-stage therapy on disease progression in AAV-mediated rescue of photoreceptor cells in the retinoschisin-deficient mouse. Molecular Therapy. 2008;**16**(6):1010-1017

[15] Pellissier LP, Hoek RM, Vos RM, Aartsen WM, Klimczak R, Hoyng S, et al. Specific tools for targeting and expression in Müller glial cells. Molecular Therapy - Methods & Clinical Development. 2014;**1**(2):14009

[16] Pellissier LP, Quinn PM, Alves CH, et al. Gene therapy into photoreceptors and Müller glial cells restores retinal structure and function in CRB1 retinitis pigmentosa mouse models. Human Molecular Genetics. 2015;**24**(2):1-15

[17] Le Meur G, Lebranchu P, Billaud F, Adjali O, Schmitt S, Bézieau S, et al. Safety and long-term efficacy of AAV4 gene therapy in patients with RPE65 Leber congenital Amaurosis. Molecular Therapy. 2018;**26**(1):256-268

[18] Weleber RG, Pennesi ME, Wilson DJ, Kaushal S, Erker LR, Jensen L, et al. Results at 2 years after gene therapy for RPE65-deficient Leber congenital Amaurosis and severe early-childhood–onset retinal dystrophy. Ophthalmology. 2016;**123**(7):1606-1620

[19] Acland GM, Aguirre GD, Bennett J, Aleman TS, Cideciyan AV, Bennicelli J, et al. Long-term restoration of rod and cone vision by single dose rAAV-mediated gene transfer to the retina in a canine model of childhood blindness. Molecular Therapy. 2005;**12**(6): 1072-1082

[20] Bainbridge JWB, Mehat MS, Sundaram V, Robbie SJ, Barker SE, Ripamonti C, et al. Long-term effect of gene therapy on Leber's congenital Amaurosis. The New England Journal of Medicine. 2015;**372**(20):1887-1897

[21] Cideciyan AV, Aleman TS, Boye SL, Schwartz SB, Kaushal S, Roman AJ, et al. Human gene therapy for RPE65 isomerase deficiency activates the retinoid cycle of vision but with slow rod kinetics. Proceedings of the National Academy of Sciences of the United States of America. 2008;**105**(39):15112-15117

[22] Maguire AM, Simonelli F, Pierce EA, Pugh EN, Mingozzi F, Bennicelli J, et al. Safety and efficacy of gene transfer for Leber's congenital amaurosis. The New England Journal of Medicine. 2008;**358**(21):2240-2248

[23] Maclachlan TK, Milton MN, Turner O, Tukov F, Choi VW, Penraat J, et al. Nonclinical safety evaluation of scAAV8-RLBP1 for treatment of RLBP1 retinitis Pigmentosa. Molecular Therapy - Methods & Clinical Development. 2018;**8**(3):105-120

[24] Pichard V, Provost N, Mendes-Madeira A, Libeau L, Hulin P, Tshilenge KT, et al. AAV-mediated gene therapy halts retinal degeneration in PDE6β-deficient dogs. Molecular Therapy. 2016;**24**(5):867-876

[25] Parinot C, Nandrot EF. A comprehensive review of mutations in the MERTK proto-oncogene. Advances in Experimental Medicine and Biology. 2016;**854**:259-265

[26] Huang WC, Wright AF, Roman AJ, Cideciyan AV, Manson FD, Gewaily DY, et al. RPGR-associated retinal degeneration in human X-linked RP and a murine model. Investigative Ophthalmology and Visual Science. 2012;**53**(9):5594-5608

[27] Beltran WA, Cideciyan AV, Lewin AS, Iwabe S, Khanna H, Sumaroka A, et al. Gene therapy rescues photoreceptor blindness in dogs and paves the way for treating human X-linked retinitis pigmentosa. Proceedings of the National Academy of Sciences of the United States of America. 2012;**109**(6):2132-2137

[28] Banin E, Gootwine E, Obolensky A, Ezra-Elia R, Ejzenberg A, Zelinger L, et al. Gene augmentation therapy restores retinal function and visual behavior in a sheep model of CNGA3 Achromatopsia. Molecular Therapy. 2015;**23**(9):1423-1433

[29] Komáromy AM, Alexander JJ, Rowlan JS, Garcia MM, Chiodo VA, Kaya A, et al. Gene therapy rescues cone function in congenital achromatopsia. Human Molecular Genetics. 2010;**19**(13):2581-2593

[30] Bush RA, Zeng Y, Colosi P, Kjellstrom S, Hiriyanna S, Vijayasarathy C, et al. Preclinical dose-escalation study of Intravitreal AAV-RS1 gene therapy in a mouse model of X-linked Retinoschisis: Dose-dependent expression and improved retinal structure and function. Human Gene Therapy. 2016;**27**(5):376-389

[31] Marangoni D, Bush RA, Zeng Y, Wei LL, Ziccardi L, Vijayasarathy C, et al. Ocular and systemic safety of a recombinant AAV8 vector for X-linked retinoschisis gene therapy: GLP studies in rabbits and Rs1-KO mice. Molecular Therapy - Methods & Clinical Development. 2016;**5**:16011

[32] Molday RS. Insights into the molecular properties of ABCA4 and its role in the visual cycle and Stargardt disease. Progress in Molecular Biology and Translational Science. 2015;**134**:415-431

[33] Koilkonda RD, Chou TH, Porciatti V, Hauswirth WW, Guy J. Induction of rapid and highly efficient expression of the human ND4 complex I subunit in the mouse visual system by self-complementary adeno-associated virus. Archives of Ophthalmology. 2010;**128**(7):876-883

[34] Vignal C, Uretsky S, Fitoussi S, Galy A, Blouin L, Girmens J-F, et al. Safety of rAAV2/2-ND4 gene therapy for Leber hereditary optic neuropathy. Ophthalmology. 2018;**S0161-6420**(17):33673-33674

[35] Cwerman-Thibault H, Augustin S, Lechauve C, Ayache J, Ellouze S, Sahel JA, et al. Nuclear expression of mitochondrial ND4 leads to the protein assembling in complex I and prevents optic atrophy and visual loss. Molecular Therapy - Methods & Clinical Development. 2015;**2**:15003

[36] Heier JS, Kherani S, Desai S, Dugel P, Kaushal S, Cheng SH, et al. Intravitreous injection of AAV2-sFLT01 in patients with advanced neovascular age-related macular degeneration: A phase 1, open-label trial. Lancet. 2017;**390**(10089):50-61

[37] Talib M, van Schooneveld MJ, van Genderen MM, Wijnholds J, Florijn RJ, ten Brink JB, et al. Genotypic and phenotypic characteristics of CRB1-associated retinal dystrophies: A long-term follow-up study. Ophthalmology. 2017;**124**(6):884-895

[38] den Hollander AI, Roepman R, Koenekoop RK, Cremers FPM. Leber congenital amaurosis: Genes, proteins and disease mechanisms. Progress in Retinal and Eye Research. 2008;**27**(4):391-419

[39] Corton M, Tatu SD, Avila-Fernandez A, Vallespín E, Tapias I, Cantalapiedra D, et al. High frequency of CRB1 mutations as cause of early-onset retinal dystrophies in the Spanish population. Orphanet Journal of Rare Diseases. 2013;**8**:20

[40] Lotery AJ, Malik A, Shami SA, Sindhi M, Chohan B, Maqbool C, et al. CRB1 mutations may result in retinitis pigmentosa without Para-arteriolar RPE preservation. Ophthalmic Genetics. 2001;**22**(3):163-169

[41] Den Hollander AI, Davis J, Van Der Velde-Visser SD, Zonneveld MN, Pierrottet CO, Koenekoop RK, et al. CRB1 mutation spectrum in inherited retinal dystrophies. Human Mutation. 2004;**24**(5):355-369

[42] Jacobson SG, Cideciyan AV, Aleman TS, Pianta MJ, Sumaroka A, Schwartz SB, et al. Crumbs homolog 1 (CRB1) mutations result in a thick human retina with abnormal lamination. Human Molecular Genetics. 2003;**12**(9):1073-1078

[43] Aleman TS, Cideciyan AV, Aguirre GK, Huang WC, Mullins CL, Roman AJ, et al. Human CRB1-associated retinal degeneration: Comparison with the rd8 Crb1-mutant mouse model. Investigative Ophthalmology and Visual Science. 2011;**52**(9):6898-6910

[44] Pellissier LP, Alves CH, Quinn PM, Vos RM, Tanimoto N, Lundvig DM, et al. Targeted ablation of Crb1 and Crb2 in retinal progenitor cells mimics Leber congenital Amaurosis. PLoS Genetics. 2013;**9**(12):e1003976

[45] Bujakowska K, Audo I, Mohand-Saïd S, Lancelot M-E, Antonio A, Germain A, et al. CRB1 mutations in inherited retinal dystrophies. Human Mutation. 2012;**33**(2):306-315

[46] Marquardt T, Gruss P. Generating neuronal diversity in the retina: One for nearly all. Trends in Neurosciences. 2002;**25**(1):32-38

[47] Alves CH, Bossers K, Vos RM, Essing AH, Swagemakers S, Van Der Spek PJ, et al. Microarray and morphological analysis of early postnatal CRB2 mutant retinas on a pure C57BL/6J genetic background. PLoS One. 2013;**8**(12):1-17

[48] Park B, Alves CH, Lundvig DM, Tanimoto N, Beck SC, Huber G, et al. PALS1 is essential for retinal pigment epithelium structure and neural retina stratification. The Journal of Neuroscience. 2011;**31**(47):17230-17241

[49] Alves CH, Sanz A, Park B, Pellissier LP, Tanimoto N, Beck SC, et al. Loss of CRB2 in the mouse retina mimics human retinitis pigmentosa due to mutations in the CRB1 gene. Human Molecular Genetics. 2013;**22**(1):35-50

[50] Alves CH, Pellissier LP, Vos RM, Garcia Garrido M, Sothilingam V, Seide C, et al. Targeted ablation of Crb2 in photoreceptor cells induces retinitis pigmentosa. Human Molecular Genetics. 2014;**23**(13):3384-3401

[51] Dudok JJ, Sanz AS, Lundvig DMS, Sothilingam V, Garrido MG, Klooster J, et al. MPP3 regulates levels of PALS1 and adhesion between photoreceptors and Müller cells. Glia. 2013;**61**(10):1629-1644

[52] van de Pavert SA, Kantardzhieva A, Malysheva A, Meuleman J, Versteeg I, Levelt C, et al. Crumbs homologue 1 is required for maintenance of photoreceptor cell polarization and adhesion during light exposure. Journal of Cell Science. 2004;**117**(18):4169-4177

[53] Tepass U, Theres C, Knust E. Crumbs encodes an EGF-like protein expressed on apical membranes of Drosophila epithelial cells and required for organization of epithelia. Cell. 1990;**61**(5):787-799

[54] Alves CH, Pellissier LP, Wijnholds J. The CRB1 and adherens junction complex proteins in retinal development and maintenance. Progress in Retinal and Eye Research. 2014;**40**:35-52

[55] Quinn PM, Pellissier LP, Wijnholds J. The CRB1 complex: Following the trail of crumbs to a feasible gene therapy strategy. Frontiers in Neuroscience. 2017;**11**(3):175

[56] Roh MH, Fan S, Liu CJ, Margolis B. The Crumbs3-Pals1 complex participates in the establishment of polarity in mammalian epithelial cells. Journal of Cell Science. 2003;**116**(14):2895-2906

[57] Kantardzhieva A, Alexeeva S, Versteeg I, Wijnholds J. MPP3 is recruited to the MPP5 protein scaffold at the retinal outer limiting membrane. The FEBS Journal. 2006;**273**(6): 1152-1165

[58] Kantardzhieva A, Gosens I, Alexeeva S, Punte IM, Versteeg I, Krieger E, et al. MPP5 recruits MPP4 to the CRB1 complex in photoreceptors. Investigative Ophthalmology and Visual Science. 2005;**46**(6):2192-2201

[59] Pellikka M, Tanentzapf G, Pinto M, Smith C, McGlade CJ, Ready DF, et al. Crumbs, the Drosophila homologue of human CRB1/RP12, is essential for photoreceptor morphogenesis. Nature. 2002;**416**(6877):143-149

[60] van Rossum AG, Aartsen WM, Meuleman J, Klooster J, Malysheva A, Versteeg I, et al. Pals1/Mpp5 is required for correct localization of Crb1 at the subapical region in polarized Müller glia cells. Human Molecular Genetics. 2006;**15**(18):2659-2672

[61] Den Hollander AI, Ghiani M, De Kok YJM, Wijnholds J, Ballabio A, Cremers FPM, et al. Isolation of Crb1, a mouse homologue of Drosophila crumbs, and analysis of its expression pattern in eye and brain. Mechanisms of Development. 2001;**110**(1-2):203-207

[62] Herranz-Martín S, Jimeno D, Paniagua AE, Velasco A, Lara JM, Aijón J, et al. Immunocytochemical evidence of the localization of the crumbs homologue 3 protein (CRB3) in the developing and mature mouse retina. PLoS One. 2012;**7**(11):e50511

[63] Quinn PM, Buck TM, Alves CH, Ohonin C, Chuva de Sousa Lopes SM, Mikkers HMM, et al. Recapitulation of the human fetal crumbs complex in human iPSCs-derived retinas and retinal pigment epithelium. Investigative Ophthalmology & Visual Science. 2017;**58**(8):3758

[64] Zhao M, Andrieu-Soler C, Kowalczuk L, Paz Cortes M, Berdugo M, Dernigoghossian M, et al. A new CRB1 rat mutation links Muller glial cells to retinal telangiectasia. The Journal of Neuroscience. 2015;**35**(15):6093-6106

[65] Aredo B, Zhang K, Chen X, Wang CX-Z, Li T, Ufret-Vincenty RLR, et al. Differences in the distribution, phenotype and gene expression of subretinal microglia/macrophages in C57BL/6N (Crb1rd8/rd8) versus C57BL6/J (Crb1wt/wt) mice. Journal of Neuroinflammation. 2015;**12**(1):6

[66] Mehalow AK, Kameya S, Smith RS, Hawes NL, Denegre JM, Young JA, et al. CRB1 is essential for external limiting membrane integrity and photoreceptor morphogenesis in the mammalian retina. Human Molecular Genetics. 2003;**12**(17):2179-2189

[67] van, de Pavert SA, Meuleman J, Malysheva A, Aartsen WM, Versteeg I, Tonagel F, et al. A single amino acid substitution (Cys249Trp) in Crb1 causes retinal degeneration and deregulates expression of pituitary tumor transforming gene Pttg1. The Journal of Neuroscience. 2007;**27**(3):564-573

[68] Naso MF, Tomkowicz B, Perry WL, Strohl WR. Adeno-associated virus (AAV) as a vector for gene therapy. BioDrugs. 2017;**31**(4):317-334

[69] Maddalena A, Tornabene P, Tiberi P, Minopoli R, Manfredi A, Mutarelli M, et al. Triple vectors expand AAV transfer capacity in the retina. Molecular Therapy. 2017:524-541

[70] Alves CH, Wijnholds J. AAV gene augmentation therapy for CRB1-associated retinitis pigmentosa. Methods in Molecular Biology. 1715;**2018**:135-151

[71] Ochakovski GA, Bartz-Schmidt KU, Fischer MD. Retinal gene therapy: Surgical vector delivery in the translation to clinical trials. Frontiers in Neuroscience. 2017;**11**:174

[72] Fischer MD, Hickey DG, Singh MS, MacLaren RE. Evaluation of an optimized injection system for retinal gene therapy in human patients. Human Gene Therapy Methods. 2016;**27**(4):150-158

[73] Du L, Peng H, Wu Q, Zhu M, Luo D, Ke X, et al. Observation of total VEGF level in hyperglycemic mouse eyes after intravitreal injection of the novel anti-VEGF drug conbercept. Molecular Vision. 2015;**21**(7):185-193

[74] Dureau P, Legat L, Neuner-Jehle M, Bonnel S, Pecqueur S, Abitbol M, et al. Quantitative analysis of subretinal injections in the rat. Graefe's Archive for Clinical and Experimental Ophthalmology. 2000;**238**:608-614

[75] Chiu K, Chang RC-C, So K-F. Intravitreous injection for establishing ocular diseases model. Journal of Visualized Experiments. 2007;**8**:313

[76] Klimczak RR, Koerber JT, Dalkara D, Flannery JG, Schaffer DV. A novel adeno-associated viral variant for efficient and selective intravitreal transduction of rat Müller cells. PLoS One. 2009;**4**(10):e7467

[77] Buck TM, Pellissier LP, Vos RM, van Dijk EHC, Boon CJF, Wijnholds J. AAV serotype testing on cultured human donor retinal explants. Methods in Molecular Biology. 1715;**2018**:275-288

[78] Orlans HO, Edwards TL, De Silva SR, Patrício MI, MacLaren RE. Human retinal explant culture for ex vivo validation of AAV gene therapy. Methods in Molecular Biology. 1715;**2018**:289-303

[79] Wiley LA, Burnight ER, Kaalberg EE, Jiao C, Riker MJ, Halder JA, et al. Assessment of Adeno-associated virus serotype tropism in human retinal explants. Human Gene Therapy. 2018;**29**(4):424-436

[80] Quinn PM, Buck TM, Ohonin C, Mikkers HMM, Wijnholds J. Production of iPS-derived human retinal organoids for use in transgene expression assays. Methods in Molecular Biology. 1715;**2018**:261-273

[81] Hickey DG, Edwards TL, Barnard AR, Singh MS, De Silva SR, McClements ME, et al. Tropism of engineered and evolved recombinant AAV serotypes in the rd1 mouse and ex vivo primate retina. Gene Therapy. 2017;**24**(12):787-800

[82] Vandenberghe LH, Bell P, Maguire AM, Xiao R, Hopkins TB, Grant R, et al. AAV9 targets cone photoreceptors in the nonhuman primate retina. PLoS One. 2013;**8**(1):e53463

[83] Boye SE, Alexander JJ, Boye SL, Witherspoon CD, Sandefer KJ, Conlon TJ, et al. The human rhodopsin kinase promoter in an AAV5 vector confers rod- and cone-specific expression in the primate retina. Human Gene Therapy. 2012;**23**(10):1101-1115

[84] Buck TM, Quinn PM, Alves CH, Van Dijk E, Ohonin C, Boon CJF, et al. Potency assay for AAV-gene vectors in human iPSCs-derived retinas and donor retinas. Investigative Ophthalmology & Visual Science. 2017;**58**(8):4093

Chapter 7

Adeno-Associated Virus (AAV)-Mediated Gene Therapy for Disorders of Inherited and Non-Inherited Origin

Indu Rajapaksha, Peter Angus and
Chandana Herath

Additional information is available at the end of the chapter

http://dx.doi.org/10.5772/intechopen.80317

Abstract

Gene therapy is a novel promising approach for treating a spectrum of inherited and non-inherited disorders by delivering therapeutic genes to specific organs or tissues. Of the viral vectors that have been used to date to deliver the genes of interest, the adeno-associated viral (AAV) vector appears to be the most safe and effective vehicle and has the ability to maintain long-term gene and protein expression following a single injection of the vector. Gene therapy studies using AAV vector have shown significant progress not only in animal models but also in human gene therapy with no known pathogenicity. While success has been achieved in gene therapy using AAV vector to deliver the target genes for inherited disorders, however, clinical trials are yet to begin to see whether gene therapy has promise for treatment of non-inherited diseases. This chapter describes AAV biology, viral structure, and cell entry mechanisms, with special emphasis on AAV tissue tropism achieved by manipulating different serotypes and capsid engineering. This chapter also discusses successful application of the AAV vector for non-inherited disorders in animal models with particular reference to liver fibrosis, outlining advantages, disadvantages, and future challenges that this therapy may face.

Keywords: adeno-associated viral vector (AAV), gene therapy, inherited disorders, non-inherited disorders, liver fibrosis

1. Introduction

Gene therapy is a novel promising approach for treating a spectrum of inherited and non-inherited disorders by delivering therapeutic genes to specific organs or tissues. Of the viral vectors that have been used to date to deliver the gene of interest, the adeno-associated viral (AAV) vector appears to be the most safe and effective vehicle and has the ability to maintain long-term gene and protein expression following a single injection of the vector. Gene therapy studies using AAV vector have shown significant progress not only in animal models but also in human gene therapy with no known pathogenicity. Recently, the Food and Drug Administration (FDA) has approved a pioneering gene therapy protocol using an AAV vector for a rare form of childhood blindness, the first such treatment cleared in the United States for an inherited disease. While success has been achieved in this field targeting inherited disorders, however, clinical trials are yet to begin to see whether gene therapy has promise for treatment of non-inherited diseases. This chapter describes AAV biology, viral structure, and cell entry mechanisms, with special emphasis on AAV tissue tropism achieved by manipulating different serotypes and capsid engineering. This chapter also discusses successful application of the AAV vector for non-inherited disorders in animal models with particular reference to liver fibrosis, outlining advantages, disadvantages, and future challenges that this therapy may face.

2. Adeno-associated virus

Adeno-associated virus (AAV) was discovered by Atchison et al. in 1965 from a pooled harvest of rhesus monkey kidney cell (RMK) cultures coinfected with simian adenovirus type 1 (SV15) [1]. This virus that could be observed as small DNA-containing particles was initially discovered as a contaminant of adenovirus preparations, and thus, it was named adeno-associated virus. However, AAV belongs to a genus of the parvoviruses, now known as dependoviruses [2]. AAV is replication defective and depends on a helper virus for effective and productive replication in mammalian cells. Generally, adenovirus or herpes viruses are considered to be the helper viruses for AAV to continue its life cycle. Early research on AAV has shown that this virus does not cause any disease in man even though it appears that it persists in humans along with its helper virus, particularly adenovirus [2]. In 1969, AAV was shown to possess several advantages in experimental systems including its small DNA genome of approximately 5 kb, packaging of plus and minus strands into individual particles, and most importantly, it is present as a defective virus [3]. During the first 20 years after its discovery, its genome structure, growth cycle, and latency were described. In the early 1980s, the genome sequencing of AAV serotype 2 (AAV2) was completed by Srivastava and colleagues [3]. This facilitated the generation of the first recombinant AAV vectors using AAV2 by the mid-1980s. Thereafter, studies using AAV were used for gene transfer in mammalian cell cultures. Subsequently, evidence of clinical safety has encouraged the researchers to use AAV vectors in clinical trials for various inherited disorders [4].

The AAV2 is a non-enveloped virion with a genome consisting of a single-stranded DNA (ssDNA) which is enclosed by a spherical protein shell about 20 nm in diameter [5, 6], with a density of 1.41 g/cm^3 [6, 7]. The AAV genome is made up of 4675 nucleotides flanked by inverted terminal repeats (ITRs). Each ITR is 145 nucleotides in length and forms a T-shaped hairpin structure by self-base pairing utilizing the first 125 nucleotides [3, 8]. Viral replication (Rep) and capsid (Cap) genes responsible for encoding four non-structural proteins, such as Rep40, Rep52, Rep68, and Rep78, and three structural proteins, such as VP1, VP2, and VP3, respectively, are located between the two ITR regions. The structural proteins, VP1, VP2, and VP3, are arranged in a ratio of 1:1:10 to form the icosahedral symmetrical shape of the virus [6, 9]. It has been reported that the VP1 protein is essential for infection [6, 10], whereas VP2 is the major protein responsible for nuclear transfer of the capsid proteins. Of note, the VP3 subunit is the most abundant protein in the capsid responsible for the binding of the virus to cell surface receptors [6, 11] and viral particle formation in the host cell [12].

3. AAV-host cell interaction

Heparan sulfate proteoglycan (HSPG) is the first identified primary receptor that AAV2 binds when infecting cells [6, 13]. The initial hypothesis was that the HSPG-binding site is located within the capsid protein VP3 [14], and this hypothesis was further supported by a mutational analysis performed by Wu and colleagues in year 2000 [11]. Wu et al. showed that there are two VP3 amino acid clusters of AAV2 that are involved in HSPG binding [11]. HSPG is not the only receptor type involved in AAV2 binding to a host cell, but there are one or more coreceptors which facilitate AAV cellular entry. Interestingly, $\alpha v\beta 5$ integrin was identified as a coreceptor for internalization of AAV2 virions by Summerford and colleagues [15]. In cell studies, the chelating agent ethylenediaminetetraacetic acid (EDTA) was used to disrupt integrin function and results showed a notable reduction in AAV2 infection, suggesting that AAV2 uses $\alpha v\beta 5$ integrin as a secondary receptor to mediate viral entry. Moreover, Qing and colleagues identified that human fibroblast growth factor receptor 1 (FGFR1) is also essential for viral entry into the host cell [16] and acts as a coreceptor for successful infection by AAV [6].

Although AAV2 is the most extensively studied serotype of AAV, there are several other AAV serotypes which have been evaluated for their binding characteristics to cellular receptors. It was recently shown that AAV serotypes 3 [17] and 13 (VR-942) [18] utilize HSPG as the primary cell surface receptor for cell entry, while AAV serotypes 1, 4, 5, and 6 [18–20] utilize N-linked and O-linked $\alpha 2$–3 and $\alpha 2$–6 sialic acids. AAV9 interacts with N-terminal galactose as the primary receptor [21] and also interacts with secondary coreceptors for facilitating cell entry, such as integrins [15, 22] FGFR1 [16], hepatocyte growth factor receptor (c-Met) [23], and laminin receptor [24]. Despite all these known pathways for AAV infection, no common primary receptor for all the AAV serotypes had been identified. Recently, Pillay and colleagues [25] used a library of mutagenized haploid HAP1 cells to create knockouts of nearly all non-essential genes in the human genome. This knockout library was exposed to recombinant AAV2-RFP (AAV2-red fluorescent protein), and a gene that was most significantly enriched in the screen was identified. This receptor named "AAV receptor (AAVR)" is characterized as a type I transmembrane protein which contains a MANSC domain, five polycystic kidney disease (PKD) domains, and a C6 region near the N terminus. These findings have been validated using an AAVR knockout cell line which demonstrated a resistant to infection by almost all AAV serotypes, whereas restoring recombinant AAVR gene in the AAVR knockout cells restored the ability of AAVs for successful infection. Furthermore, AAVR gene knockout mice demonstrated robust resistance to AAV9 infection. This important discovery implicates the AAVR as a universal primary receptor for all AAV serotype infection [6].

4. Cell entry mechanism of AAV

The major cell entry mechanism for AAV is via endocytosis utilizing clathrin-coated pits, although other minor mechanisms are possibly involved in this process. However, these alternative minor mechanisms are yet to be confirmed [6]. Upon AAV binding to its cell surface receptors, it stimulates intracellular signaling pathways, which in turn stimulates internalization of AAV. This phenomenon can be clearly explained using the mechanisms reported for AAV2 host cell interaction. It was shown that attachment of AAV2 to HSPG and $\alpha V\beta 5$ integrin resulted in the activation of Rac1, an intracellular small guanosine triphosphate (GTP)-binding protein, and phosphoinositide 3-kinase (PI3K) in HeLa cells within 5 minutes of AAV2 infection [26]. Furthermore, inhibition of Notch1 by siRNA, a transmembrane receptor known to be involved in the activation of Rac1 and PI3K, was reported to decrease cell transduction by AAV2 [27], suggesting that the Rac1-PI3K pathway is necessary to initiate endocytosis of AAV2. Direct injection of AAV into the cytoplasm and nucleus of cells results in a significant lower infection rate than cells that are simply exposed to virus [28], suggesting that the processing of AAV virion through endosomal compartments is a critical initiating step for transduction following endocytosis.

In addition, transduction efficiency of AAV is largely dependent on the endosomal pH. Changing the pH to acidic (pH 4–6) inside the endosomal compartment facilitates transduction of AAV, whereas blocking acidification during endosomal processing decreases the rate of transduction [29–31]. Also, the application of different classes of proteasome inhibitors such as tripeptidyl aldehydes and N-acetyl-L-leucyl-L-leucyl-L-norleucinal (LLnL) and the anthracycline compounds such as doxorubicin increases the rate of viral translocation to the nucleus [32]. Furthermore, LLnL appears to increase AAV2 capsid ubiquitination that results in augmented gene transfer in different cell types [33], suggesting a mechanism by which these inhibitors increase transduction may be related to ubiquitination. AAV must exit from the endosome first before translocating to the nucleus. Prior to escape from the endosome, AAV undergoes a conformational change leading to the exposure of the unique N-terminal ends of VP1 and VP2, which contains a domain of phospholipase A2 (PLA2) [34], an enzyme that breaches the endosomal membrane and thereby facilitates efficient endosomal escape of viral particles. Upon endosomal escape, AAV enters the nucleus as an intact particle [28] and uncoating then occurs inside the nucleus. However, nuclear transport of AAV is a slow process, approximately only 1–2% of internalized AAV enters and expresses in the nucleus, and the whole entry process takes about 2–13 h [35]. Thus, most viral particles which fail to translocate are located outside or away from the nucleus.

The viral particles that fail to translocate into the nucleus are eventually degraded by host proteasomes in the cytoplasm and presented as antigen to cytotoxic T cells via the major histocompatibility complex (MHC) class I pathway [36]. Although there are several studies that have investigated the nuclear entry of AAV, the mechanism by which AAV translocates into the nucleus is still unclear. Because AAV is a small virus with a diameter of around 20 nm, it has been suggested that the virion enters the nucleus using the nuclear pore complex (NPC) [37].

Furthermore, the nuclear entry of AAV is dependent on importin-β, a nuclear import protein that has been shown to play a key role in facilitating the binding of viral particles to host nuclei in other viral infectious pathways [38, 39]. Another study using single-point edge excitation sub-diffraction (SPEED) microscopy, a form of super-resolution imaging, to track single AAV particles revealed that approximately 17% of AAV particles were imported through the NPC successfully to the nucleus [40], reinforcing the importance of the NPC in AAV nuclear transfer. Interestingly, there is further evidence that nucleolin, a protein that shuttles between cytoplasm and nucleus, specifically binds to AAV capsid, which suggests that nucleolin may act as a nuclear receptor for AAV particles as well [41]. Upon entry into the nucleus, the ssDNA of AAV genome is converted to double-stranded DNA (dsDNA) using nuclear machinery of the target cells for transcription of the transgene [42]. The synthesis of second DNA strand has been considered as a rate-limiting factor for the onset and efficiency of transgene expression in ssAAV vectors [43]. As a result, second-generation AAV vectors with a dsDNA, also known as self-complementary AAV (scAAV) vectors, have been developed to improve the transduction and transcription efficiency. In the past decade, several studies have shown that new scAAV vectors provide safe, reliable, and organ-specific transduction both *in vitro* [44–46] and *in vivo* [46–49]. This suggests that the limitations associated with cell transduction using ssAAV genome can be overcome by the use of scAAV vectors in gene therapy.

5. AAV serotypes and tissue tropism

To date, a total of 12 naturally occurring AAV serotypes have been discovered from both human and non-human primates (**Table 1**). These serotypes are able to infect cells of diverse tissue types. Interestingly, the tissue specificity is determined by the capsid serotype. The existence of a variety of serotypes with different infectivity rates and tissue specificity makes AAV one of the most promising candidates in gene therapy research. By development of different AAV pseudotypes, researchers have been able to obtain unique cellular tropism and high transduction efficiency. All AAV serotypes share at least 50% sequence homology. However, serotype AAV5 has the most divergent amino acid capsid sequence, and AAV4 also shows a considerable degree of divergence [50]. Surprisingly, this sequence diversity between serotypes is not scattered but primarily located in the looped out domains of the capsid protein [51]. However, comparative studies of AAV serotypes found that this sequence variability may not be responsible for the differences in infectivity rates and tissue specificity. AAV serotype 2 is most widely used in gene therapy research. Several studies have investigated gene expression and tropism *in vivo* mediated by different AAV serotypes and identified that they differ broadly in transduction efficacies and tissue tropism. A comparative study of AAV serotypes 1–9 mediated transgene expression after systemic

AAV serotype	Characteristics	Tissue tropism
AAV1	Shares 99% homology with AAV6 serotype [50]	Liver, heart, skeletal muscle [52]
AAV2	The most commonly used serotype Close homology to all serotypes except AAV 4, 5, 11, and 12 [50] Low transduction efficiency [52]	Liver, heart, muscle [52]
AAV3	Low transduction efficiency Slow in targeting the tissues [52]	Heart, liver [52]
AAV4	Close homology to AAV11 (82%) and AAV12 (79%) serotypes [50] Low transduction efficiency Slow in targeting the tissues [52]	Lung, heart, liver, central nervous system [52, 134]
AAV5	The most divergent serotype (shares only 53–59% homology to other serotypes) Low transduction efficiency [52]	Liver [52]
AAV6	Shares 99% homology with AAV1 serotype [50]	Liver, heart, skeletal muscle [52]
AAV7	Fast in targeting the tissues [52]	Liver, skeletal muscle [52]
AAV8	93% homology to AAV10 serotype [50]	Heart, liver, brain, muscle (second most efficient serotype reaching the brain) [52]
AAV9	Fast in targeting the tissues [52]	Liver, heart, brain, lung, skeletal muscle (serotype with the broadest tissue tropism and most efficient in reaching the brain) [52]
AAV10	93% homology to AAV8 serotype [50]	Liver, heart, muscle, lung, kidney, uterus (with pseudotype AAV2/10) [135]
AAV11	Close homology to AAV4 serotype [50]	Muscle, kidney, spleen, lung, heart, stomach (with pseudotype AAV2/11) [135]
AAV12	Close homology to AAV4 serotype [50]	Muscle, salivary glands [136]

Table 1. Characteristics and tissue tropism of AAV serotypes in the mouse.

tail vein injection in mice showed that each AAV serotype profoundly differs in its ability to transduce organs, with AAV9 having the highest and fastest onset of transgene expression, highest viral genome copies, and the broadest tissue tropism, as determined by luciferase images [52]. Conversely, AAV3 and AAV4 are the slowest in targeting tissues, and among all the serotypes, AAV2, 3, 4, and 5 have the lowest transduction efficiency. The liver is the most common organ transduced by nearly all AAV serotypes with AAV7 and AAV9 showing the strongest tropism. Moreover, AAV9 is the most efficient serotype in reaching the heart and brain, followed by AAV4 and AAV8, respectively [52]. Of note, AAV serotype 8 (AAV8) shows a significantly greater liver transduction efficiency than the other AAV serotypes, and therefore, this serotype has been developed to use as a gene therapy vector for hemophilia A and familial hypercholesterolemia [53].

6. Molecular engineering of AAV capsid

There are several challenges for AAV serotypes to exert their therapeutic potential in target organs including the need for high vector doses for efficient delivery, pre-existing antiviral immunity in the host, and the lack of cell type-specific tropism leading to off-target transduction [6]. One way to overcome these limitations is to randomly generate capsid mutants from a library to extend the capability of the traditional AAV vector by increasing its cell transduction efficiency for specific cell types and its ability to escape from antibody neutralization.

One approach used to create a mutant library is DNA shuffling, a strategy in which the open reading frame of capsid genes of different AAV serotypes is fragmented by nucleases. This is followed by random ligation, resulting in new and random combinations of capsid sequences. These new molecular-enhanced AAV vectors exhibit a broad range of cell tropism with numerous functional differences between chimeras and their parent serotypes. Consequently, there is potential to produce unlimited numbers of new AAV variants with novel gene delivery properties. This method of AAV capsid engineering was first described in 2008 by Grimm and colleagues [54] and has become a commonly used technique over the years. More recently, Lisowski and colleagues utilized a humanized mouse model to perform serial selection using a human-specific replication competent viral library composed of DNA-shuffled AAV capsids. After four rounds of selection, they identified a novel chimeric capsid variant composed of five different parental AAV capsids [55]. Of these, LK-03, which efficiently transduced human primary hepatocytes both *in vitro* and *in vivo*, was found to be a human liver cell-specific AAV serotype [55]. This study has opened up a new avenue to validate therapeutic potential of an AAV capsid variant in preclinical studies using human primary cell xenotransplanted models prior to commencing clinical studies.

In addition, a study using *in silico* ancestral sequence reconstruction (ASR) of AAV capsid protein generated nine functional putative ancestral AAVs. In this study, Zinn and colleagues also identified Anc80, the predicted ancestral sequence of the widely used AAV serotypes 1, 2, 8, and 9 and showed that Anc80 is a highly potent *in vivo* gene therapy vector compared to AAV2 and AAV8 for targeting liver, muscle, and retina in mice [56]. Nevertheless, Anc80 demonstrated a high stability and no toxicity in several safety studies carried out in mice. This synthetic viral vector has been evaluated in non-human primates (rhesus macaques), which demonstrated a superior expression of Anc80 in monkey liver following Anc80 administration compared to control monkeys injected with AAV8. Hence, future studies may also rely on the use of Anc80, in particular for liver-directed gene therapy studies.

7. AAV as a safe vector in gene therapy

It has been shown that AAV viral proteins cause a minimal immunogenic response, and at the same time, it can yield prolonged expression of therapeutically relevant genes/proteins. Also, when comparing to the other potential viral vectors such as lentiviral vectors, AAV possesses a reduced proinflammatory risk and has been considered as one of the most promising gene transfer vectors for *in vivo* gene therapy [57]. However, in some experimental settings, it was reported that immune responses generated by AAV administration appear to compromise the outcomes of AAV-mediated gene therapy. Thus, several factors may determine the occurrence of immune responses against the AAV proteins, including the route of administration, dose, serotype, host species, transgene and expression cassettes, and pre-existing immunity to AAV [6, 58].

It has been suggested that AAV activates mouse and human plasmacytoid DCs to produce type 1 interferon via a TLR9-MyD88 pathway, resulting in induction of adaptive immune CD8+ T cell responses to AAV capsid and the transgene [58]. In addition, different administration routes for AAV2-mediated ocular gene therapy induced varying immune responses. For instance, intravitreal administration of an AAV2 vector, which led to transduction of the inner retina, triggered a humoral immune response to AAV2 capsid; however, no effect was observed following subretinal administration and subsequent repeated injections [59]. Animal studies have suggested that the presence of neutralizing antibodies could compromise AAV transduction *in vivo* following systemic administration [60, 61]. These findings are potentially important for translation of AAV gene therapy from animal studies to clinical trials due to the large prevalence of AAV neutralizing antibodies in humans.

Due to natural exposure to wild-type AAV early in life, a significant proportion of human population have humoral immunity to the AAV capsid, primarily AAV1, 2, 3, and 5 [62, 63]. Of note, among the most commonly used AAV vectors, the most prevalent anti-AAV antibodies in humans are AAV2 followed by anti-AAV antibodies to AAV1 [64], while the least prevalent are for AAV7 and AAV8. It has been shown that rAAV vectors, including serotypes 1, 2, and 5 can transduce dendritic cells (DCs) and generate immune responses to transgene products [65, 66]. Interestingly, another study, which evaluated the differential immune responses to the transgene products from rAAV1 and rAAV8 vectors using a hypersensitive autoimmune mouse model, revealed that unlike AAV1 vectors, AAV8 vectors were unable to transduce dendritic cells (DCs) and elicit transgene-specific immune responses efficiently, resulting in induction of immune tolerance to transgene products [67]. Different properties of these vectors imply tremendous potential in different applications, where an immune response to transgene is to be either elicited or avoided.

8. AAV vector transduction efficiency—male versus female

Recombinant AAV vector transduction efficiency clearly depends on the gender. This fact has been specifically shown in the liver and the brain in murine models. A study carried out by Maguire and colleagues has shown that the vector transduction efficiency using AAV serotype 9 was found to be different in the brain and the liver between male and female mice [68]. This study revealed a higher transgene expression in the brain of females compared with male mice, whereas a higher transgene expression was observed in the liver of male mice compared with female mice. In line with this study, Davidoff and colleagues revealed that when compared with female mice, transgene expression after liver-targeted delivery of AAV2 and AAV5 particles was 5- to 13-fold higher in male mice [69]. In addition, they found that transduction efficiency was dramatically reduced by castration in male mice, whereas oophorectomy in female mice did not significantly influence rAAV transduction [69]. Moreover, administration of 5α dihydrotestosterone in female mice prior to rAAV injection enhanced stable hepatocyte gene transfer to levels observed in male mice, suggesting rAAV vector transduces hepatocytes via an androgen-dependent pathway [69].

In addition, there is evidence to demonstrate the distinctly different patterns of persistence of rAAV-eGFP (enhanced green fluorescent protein) expression across the hepatic lobule in male and female mice. Female mice retained a predominantly perivenous pattern of expression, whereas male mice had shown an inversion of this pattern with preferential loss of perivenous expression and relative retention of periportal expression [70]. Therefore, these sexually dimorphic patterns of genome persistence could have significant implications for the long-term therapeutic efficacy of rAAV-mediated gene transfer in man, particularly in the context of correction of liver functions showing metabolic zonation [70].

9. Production and modification of AAV

The AAV serotype 2 was the first AAV vector used for gene transfer applications. This particular vector was chosen primarily because of its broad tropism, efficient transduction with stable and long-term transgene expression with minimal inflammation, and immune responses in a number of organs, such as the brain [71], retina [72], and skeletal muscles [73]. Liver is the other major organ which is targeted for rAAV2 gene delivery strategy because hepatocytes are easily accessible to vectors injected into the circulation through large pores in liver capillaries. Although results in the liver have been less consistent, a number of studies demonstrate a successful transduction of rAAV2 vector with persistent transgene expression in the liver using a single dose [74], and approximately 5% of hepatocytes were transduced following rAAV2 vector injection [75]. Of note, a study which was undertaken by Snyder and colleagues provided the most impressive results by achieving sustained and therapeutic levels of factor IX in hemophilia B, with no associated toxicity in both canine and murine models [75, 76].

The discovery of novel strategies for pseudotyping, recombination of AAV constructs into capsids of alternative serotypes, and the development of scAAV vectors which effectively alter tissue tropisms with enhanced transduction efficiency [77] has opened up new avenues to produce more attractive vectors for use in clinical applications including hemophilia B, Parkinson's disease, and rheumatoid arthritis [78]. Among all novel recombinant AAV serotypes, AAV2 genome construct pseudotyped with capsid 8 (AAV2/8) is one of the most efficient vectors for hepatic gene transfer. In addition, it has greater liver transduction efficiency, with fourfold more genomes per transduced cell, when compared with other pseudotyped vectors [6, 79]. Moreover, it has an excellent transduction rate (95%) in hepatocytes of the mouse liver via intraportal vein injection [80]. In line with this, the development of scAAV vectors further enhances the transduction efficiency to the liver [81], suggesting that the conversion of single-stranded AAV genome into double-stranded form for gene therapy studies appears to be beneficial since this procedure can avoid the need to assemble second DNA strand for transgene expression *in vivo* [6, 46, 82].

The most widely used method to produce and purify recombinant AAV particles for preclinical applications is the triple transfection method using HEK293 cells, which requires the use of an

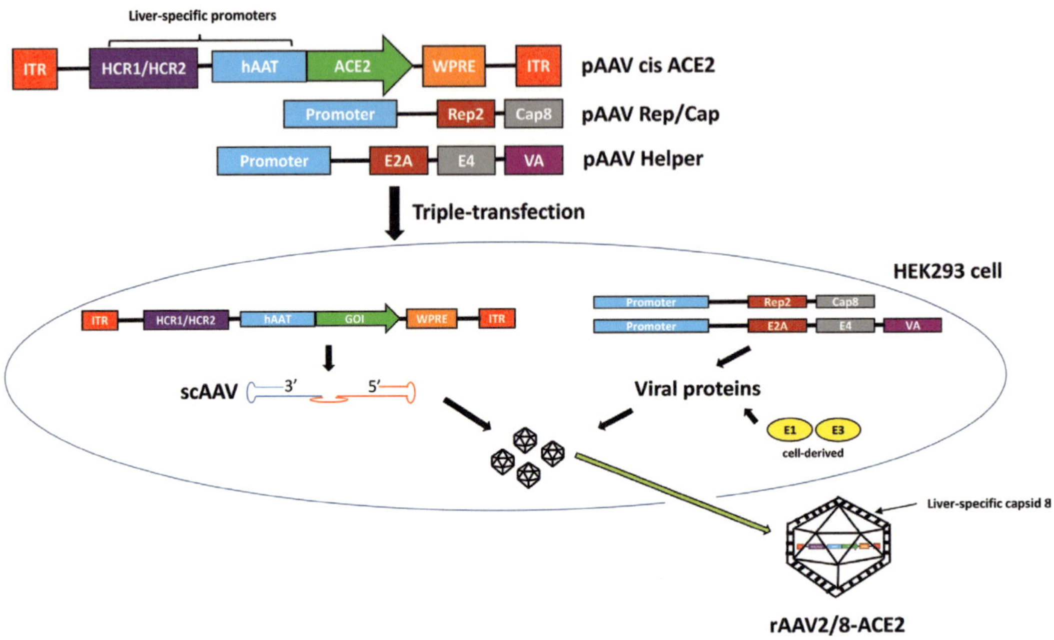

Figure 1. Schematic representation of the assembly of AAV2 genome pseudotyped with liver-specific AAV serotype 8 and liver-specific promoters in HEK293 cells. Liver-specific rAAV2/8-ACE2 viral particles are produced by transfecting HEK293 cells with rep2/cap8 plasmid, Ad helper plasmid, and a plasmid carrying AAV2 inverted terminal repeat-ACE2 cassette with liver-specific promoters. Recombinant AAV2/8-ACE2 viral particles are purified from cell homogenate 48–72 h post transfection, followed by assessment of AAV quality, genome titer, infectious and transducing properties, and integrity of the packaged AAV genome [87].

AAV replication and capsid plasmid that provides Rep78, Rep68, Rep52, and Rep40 proteins necessary for vector genome replication and VP1, VP2, and VP3 capsid proteins, the vector DNA plasmid with the inverted terminal repeat-transgene cassette, as well as the adenovirus (Ad) helper plasmid [83, 84]. In addition, HEK293 cells have been engineered to provide adenovirus helper genes *in trans* such as E1a and E1b55k for AAV assembly. The key advantage of this method is that AAV particles can be efficiently made with genes supplied by Ad helper and HEK293 cells without the need to use replication competent adenovirus [84] (**Figure 1**). In addition, to improve tissue tropism, the AAV genomes can be pseudotyped with a desired capsid protein. Following 48–72 h transfection, the cell homogenate is purified, followed by the assessment of AAV quality control including genome titer [85], infectious and transducing properties, and integrity of the packaged AAV genome [86]. This is schematically illustrated in **Figure 1** where AAV2 genome is pseudotyped with capsid 8 (AAV2/8) to increase liver specificity [87].

10. Pros and cons of AAV gene therapy

A successful gene therapy approach should deliver an appropriate amount of a therapeutic gene into the target tissue without substantial toxicity while achieving long-term gene expression. Of all currently available viral vectors including retroviral, lentiviral, adenoviral, and AAV vectors, the AAV is a unique non-pathogenic viral vector with broad tissue tropism and has the potential

http://dx.doi.org/10.5772/intechopen.80317

to be the leading vector for future gene therapy studies [88]. Unlike recombinant adenoviral vectors which yield high initial gene expression that diminishes rapidly due to immune clearance, the AAV vector-based gene expression is persistent. In addition, as AAV vectors were derived from a parental virus with no known pathogenesis which is replication defective, they do not carry a risk of infecting patients with a pathogenic wild type virus. In addition, AAV vectors mediate a minimal cell-mediated immune response, which is favorable for the persistence gene transduction to the host cells. At the same time, AAV-based vectors are able to transduce a wide range of host cells including both dividing and non-dividing cell types [88, 89]. A prominent disadvantage associated with AAV compared to the other viral vectors is its small packaging size, which limits the size of the transgene to be delivered using the vector. However, novel molecular engineering methods have the potential to overcome these limitations, and thus, genetically engineered AAV is poised to become the leading vector for future gene therapy in humans.

11. Gene therapy using AAV vectors for inherited disorders

Many studies have explored the therapeutic potential of these engineered AAV vectors for a number of inherited disorders. After several decades of experimental studies, the first successful human gene therapy protocol using AAV serotype 1 vector was approved in 2012 by the European Commission (EU) for the treatment of patients with lipoprotein lipase deficiency (LPLD), an extremely rare genetic disorder [90]. This was a milestone achievement for researchers who have been working to develop successful gene therapy protocols for inherited human disorders. The therapy was introduced under the trade name Glybera® (alipogene tiparvovec) by UniQure. However, after 5 years of the launch of the world's first approved gene therapy, UniQure has not renewed its EU license in 2017 and ceased to produce Glybera for use because of the expensive nature of the treatment protocol [91]. However, it was unfortunate that UniQure has discontinued its production despite the first LPLD patient treated with alipogene tiparvovec showing improvement of quality of life without abdominal pain and pancreatitis attacks for 18 months [92]. UniQure, however, has endeavored to develop gene therapy for hemophilia B.

The most common clinical trials based on AAV therapy in recent years have been in hemophilia B, a blood clotting disorder caused by a defect in the gene encoding coagulation Factor IX (FIX), leading to a deficiency of FIX. The only treatment available for this disease is lifelong intravenous infusion of FIX concentrates. Although this treatment is effective as a preventive medicine, it is not curative. In addition, the treatment is invasive, inconvenient, and very expensive, thus not affordable for most patients with hemophilia B, resulting in a reduction in life expectancy for those patients with a severe bleeding phenotype [93]. Similar to the FIX concentrates, there are clotting formulations with longer half-life which represents a major advance but still require lifelong intravenous administration. Robust preclinical results using AAV-based therapy in two murine [74, 94] and three canine models of hemophilia B [95–97] demonstrated long-term expression of FIX, with no significant liver toxicity and with no FIX-specific antibodies detected following muscle- or liver-directed injections. A follow-up study demonstrated an induction of immune tolerance in mice after hepatic gene transfer by rAAV expressing human FIX (rAAV-hFIX), which is mediated by regulatory CD4+ T cells, resulting in suppression of human FIX antibody formation [6, 98]. Based on the results from animal studies, the world first clinical trial using rAAV2-hFIX vector in humans via intramuscular route has been conducted [99]. The results indicated that the transduction of muscle tissue was successful; however, circulating plasma FIX levels in all patients were less than the required level for a therapeutic effect (<2% of normal). In a subsequent clinical study, the delivery target was switched to the liver, the normal site of FIX synthesis. Although rAAV2-mediated hFIX gene transfer to the liver-mediated therapeutically relevant expression levels [100], the expression persisted for less than 8 weeks.

Recent study by Nathwani and colleagues demonstrated the AAV8 serotype as a more effective vector for liver-directed hemophilia B gene therapy [101]. In this study, six severe hemophilia B patients received a single injection of pseudotyped AAV2/8-hFIX vector at three escalating doses (high, intermediate and low), with two patients per dose and no immunosuppressive was given. Patients were subsequently followed for up to 16 months. All patients have achieved AAV2/8-mediated expression of FIX at above the therapeutic threshold, ranging between 2 and 11% of normal levels, and the increase in FIX serum level was dose-dependent. Four out of six patients discontinued their prophylactic treatment with hFIX concentrates without having spontaneous hemorrhage, whereas the other two patients continued to receive hFIX concentrates but extended the interval between hFIX treatments. This was the first liver-directed AAV gene therapy trial to show sustained therapeutic FIX levels and improved clinical outcomes in patients with hemophilia B. However, in patients who received the highest dose of vector, T cell-mediated clearance of AAV-transduced hepatocytes was observed, with associated elevation of liver enzyme levels. This response has been overcome by a short course of glucocorticoids, without the loss of hFIX expression.

Nathwani and colleagues later conducted a follow-up study to evaluate the long-term safety and efficacy of AAV2/8-hFIX therapy in the same cohort of hemophilia B patients [93]. Of note, this monitoring study also included addition of four new patients, each of whom received the high dose of vector. Consistent with their previous findings, a single intravenous injection of vector resulted in an increase in plasma FIX activity from less than 1% to sustained level of up to 6% of the normal value in all 10 patients, and this remained stable for up to a period of 4 years. Additionally, substantial clinical improvements were achieved in all patients, including significant reductions in number of spontaneous hemorrhage and annual number of prophylactic treatment with FIX concentrates. Not surprisingly, there was a dose-dependent, asymptomatic increase in both the serum alanine transaminase (ALT) level and increase in anti-AAV capsid neutralizing antibody level, which led to a gradual decline in FIX levels, suggesting transduced hepatocyte destruction. There was a transient increase of ALT levels in all patients which resolved with administration of a single course of prednisolone, after which no recurrent elevation of serum ALT in patients was observed.

A recent clinical trial completed using ssAAV vector consisted of a bioengineered capsid, liver-specific promoter, and FIX Padua (FIX-R338L) in 10 men with hemophilia B who had FIX coagulant activity of 2% or less of the normal also showed a success with no serious adverse events during or after vector infusion [102]. These patients were followed up to 492 days (16 months). The results showed that 8 of 10 patients did not require the regular treatment with FIX concentrates, and bleeding episodes were not reported in 9 patients after the vector treatment. Overall, there was a significant reduction in annual bleeding rate in patients treated with AAV-FIX-R338L. Although there were two patients who developed asymptomatic increase in liver enzyme levels, they were recovered after a short-term prednisone treatment. Of all participants, only one patient had been treated with FIX concentrates who was diagnosed with an advanced arthropathy at baseline. However, the use of FIX concentrate was reduced to 91% comparing to the status before vector infusion. Additional clinical trials are underway with AAV2/8-hFIX (NCT00979238) and FIX-Padua (NCT01687608), which will provide more information on safety and efficacy of the therapy [103]. Overall, the results from these studies suggest that gene therapy has the potential to significantly improve disease phenotype in hemophilia B patients.

It is of significance that for the first time, the US Food and Drug Administration (FDA) has approved a pioneering gene therapy protocol using an AAV vector for a rare form of childhood blindness in 2017 as the first such treatment cleared in the United States for an inherited disease. The disease known as Leber congenital amaurosis (LCA) develops due to mutations in the RPE65 (retinal pigment epithelium-specific 65-kDa) gene, causing a severe form of inherited retinal blindness in infants and children. Several independent studies [104–106] using rAAV2/2 expressing RPE65 complementary DNA (cDNA) have provided preliminary evidence of short-term safety and efficacy in this disorder. Further studies by Cideciyan and colleagues showed a significant efficacy of human retinal gene transfer with rAAV2-RPE65 vector with transgene expression for up to 1 year post treatment [107]. Also, they have proven the treatment as a safe therapy by evaluating the safety parameters obtained through regular standard eye examinations, physical examinations, routine hematology, serum chemistries, coagulation parameters, and urinalysis. This particular FDA-approved gene therapy (LUXTURNA) (voretigene neparvovec-rzyl) is to be used in patients with confirmed biallelic RPE65 mutation-associated retinal dystrophy. This approval is considered as a milestone of AAV vector-associated gene therapy research and further encourages researchers to develop successful vectors to deliver therapeutic genes for number of diseases where there is no effective medical treatment.

12. Gene therapy for non-inherited disorders

There have been many advances in identification of the mechanisms involved in chronic organ damage which opened up avenues for gene therapy studies [108]. While a plethora of preclinical and clinical studies over past several decades has focused on developing gene therapy for inherited disorders, despite several preclinical studies in animal models, there have been only a few clinical trials that have been undertaken to investigate therapeutic efficacy of gene therapy for non-inherited diseases. A recent study shows that telomerase expression using AAV9 vectors exerts therapeutic effects in a mouse model of pulmonary fibrosis [109]. This therapy targeted idiopathic pulmonary fibrosis. It is known that telomeres act as protective structures at the ends of chromosomes and the presence of short telomeres has been shown to be one of the causes for disease development. In this condition, telomeres become too short, resulting in the cessation of cell division which in turn leads to cell apoptosis. Telomerase is an enzyme that can restructure the telomeres length, and Povedano and colleagues developed a treatment using AAV serotype 9 to deliver telomerase to correct the short telomeres. As AAV9 preferentially targets regenerative alveolar type II cells (ATII), AAV9-Tert-treated mice show improved lung function with reduced inflammation and fibrosis at 1–3 weeks after vector treatment. It is of interest to note that pulmonary fibrosis either improved or disappeared at 8 weeks of gene therapy. AAV9-Tert treatment lead to longer telomeres and increased proliferation of ATII cells, as well as lower DNA damage, apoptosis, and senescence.

AAV vector-derived cardiac gene therapy is emerging as an entirely new platform to treat cardiac disorders [110]. AAV gene therapy for heart failure have been validated in preclinical studies using animal models, and the vast majority of these approaches have been undertaken to improve calcium handling by cardiomyocytes. The therapeutic protein used in the majority of these studies was sarcoplasmatic calcium ATPase (SERCA2a). Based on the positive preclinical findings, the first clinical trial (CUPID trial: calcium upregulation by percutaneous administration of gene vector in cardiac disease, NCT02346422) was carried out to deliver SERCA2a using AAV serotype 1 vector to treat patients with advanced heart failure [111, 112]. The outcome of this phase 1 trial was successful with no adverse events and was progressed to phase 2a study, providing promising outcomes with significantly low rate of adverse events. However, the results of phase 2b clinical trial (CUPID2b trial, NCT01643330) using the same vector were disappointing with no significant change between the treatment group and the placebo group [113]. This has led to the cessation of patient recruitment for two additional trials using AAV1. SERCA2a [110]. Interestingly, there are two new upcoming trials aimed to deliver S100A1 with an AAV9 vector and a constitutively active form of the protein phosphatase 1 inhibitors, I1c, with a chimeric capsid with AAV2 and AAV8 serotypes [114, 115]. In addition, AAV1, AAV6, and AAV9 have emerged as the most promising AAV serotypes for cardiac gene transfer, which provides hopes for successful gene therapy approaches to treat heart failure in the future.

AAV-mediated gene therapy approaches to treat neuropathic pain in rodents have also been reported [116]. Fischer and colleagues have shown that administration of rAAV expressing Ca^{2+} channel-binding domain 3 (CBD3) gene significantly reduced pain behavior such as hyperalgesia after touch with a pin or sensitivity to acetone stimulation in animal models of inflammatory and neuropathic pain [117]. Another study using AAV9 vector encoding short hairpin RNA (shRNA) against vanilloid receptor 1 (TRPV1), which is an important target gene for acute pain, demonstrated that the therapy attenuated nerve injury-induced thermal allodynia (increased response of neurons) 10–28 days after treatment in a mouse model of spared nerve injury (SNI) [118]. These results provide positive evidence to encourage gene therapy researchers to develop AAV vector-based treatments for patients with chronic/diabetic neuropathic pain.

Considerable progress has been made in gene therapy approach to treat chronic liver fibrosis. Although angiotensin-converting enzyme (ACE) inhibitors or angiotensin receptor blockers (ARBs) are widely used as treatments in patients with hypertension, they have been trialed in patients with chronic liver disease; however, the outcomes were not convincing mainly because they produce adverse systemic side effects [119]. Because of the lack of medical treatments, liver transplantation has inevitably become the only option for patients with end stage liver disease, resulting from chronic hepatic fibrosis and/or cirrhosis. Moreover, increasing incidence of chronic liver disease, lack of donor organs, post-transplantation complications, and the high cost in liver transplantation mean that there is a major need to discover and formulate specific, effective, safe, and inexpensive novel therapies for liver fibrosis/cirrhosis.

One possible approach to circumvent this is to develop organ-targeted antifibrotic strategies. Studies from our laboratory suggested that one possible target is the "alternate axis" of the renin-angiotensin system (RAS), comprising its key enzyme angiotensin-converting enzyme

2 (ACE2), which breaks down the potent profibrotic octapeptide, angiotensin II (Ang II) to an antifibrotic heptapeptide, angiotensin-(1–7) (Ang-(1–7)) [120, 121]. Evidence from experimental animal studies showed that recombinant human ACE2 (rhACE2) is beneficial for prevention of hypertension in cardiovascular disease [122] and to improve kidney function in diabetic nephropathy [123]. Interestingly, rhACE2 was well tolerated by a group of healthy human volunteers in a phase 1 clinical trial, without exerting any unwanted cardiovascular side effects [124]. There is one study that reported therapeutic effects of recombinant ACE2 in experimental liver fibrosis, in which liver injury was surgically induced by cholestasis or by hepatotoxic carbon tetrachloride injection [125]. They demonstrated that recombinant ACE2 significantly reduced hepatic fibrosis in both animal models of liver disease [125]. However, a major drawback of this systemic approach is that the treatment inevitably produces off-target effects, which in many cases are undesirable. Thus, there are several disadvantages with systemic administration of recombinant ACE2. This includes daily injections of ACE2, a procedure that is invasive in a clinical setting and expensive approach with unwanted effect on blood pressure regulation [125, 126]. To circumvent this problem, an ideal approach would be to increase tissue-specific ACE2 levels in the target organ. Thus, organ-specific increased ACE2 activity using a liver-specific recombinant AAV vector is expected to produce therapeutic effects confined to the targeted organ while minimizing unwanted off-target effects.

In addition to the use of liver-specific capsid serotype, specificity can be further enhanced by engineering the vector with ACE2 gene under the transcriptional control of a strong liver-specific promoter, apolipoprotein E/human α1-antitrypsin. Studies published by our laboratory used a pseudotyped liver-specific AAV vector (rAAV2/8) for preclinical evaluation and found that hepatic overexpression of murine ACE2 gene delivered into the mice lasted for up to 6 months following a single intraperitoneal injection [87]. We then treated mice with a range of liver disease models, which included biliary fibrosis induced by bile duct ligation (BDL), toxic injury induced by carbon tetrachloride (CCl4) injections, and fatty liver-associated liver fibrosis induced by feeding methionine- and choline-deficient (MCD) diet using a single intraperitoneal injection of rAAV2/8-ACE2 [87]. The treatment produced a major increase in ACE2 expression and protein activity, which was confined to the liver without affecting other major organs. Unlike inherited disorders, for example, hemophilia B where a relatively low level of transgene expression in the liver may be sufficient for subsequent small increases in FIX levels in the blood [48, 81], the magnitude of the expression of transgene required for therapeutic intervention in non-inherited disease may be substantially higher. This, in turn, may pose a challenge for gene therapy researchers. Interestingly, however in our liver-targeted therapeutic approach with rAAV2/8-ACE2, we found that increased hepatic ACE2 expression reduced hepatic level of profibrotic Ang II by more than 50% compared to those treated with a control vector that carried human serum albumin (rAAV2/8-HSA) [87]. A reduction of Ang II, which was accompanied by increases in hepatic levels of antifibrotic Ang-(1–7) peptide, resulted in a marked reduction in inflammatory cytokine expression, leading to a profound reduction in hepatic fibrosis in all three models (**Figure 2**) [87]. These studies with short-term animal models have been further validated to provide evidence that in long-term animal models of biliary fibrosis and fatty liver disease, which produce hepatic lesions more comparable to those seen in patients with such diseases, a single intraperitoneal injection of rAAV2/8-ACE2 caused a profound reduction in hepatic fibrosis (**Figure 3**). In marked contrast to other studies using

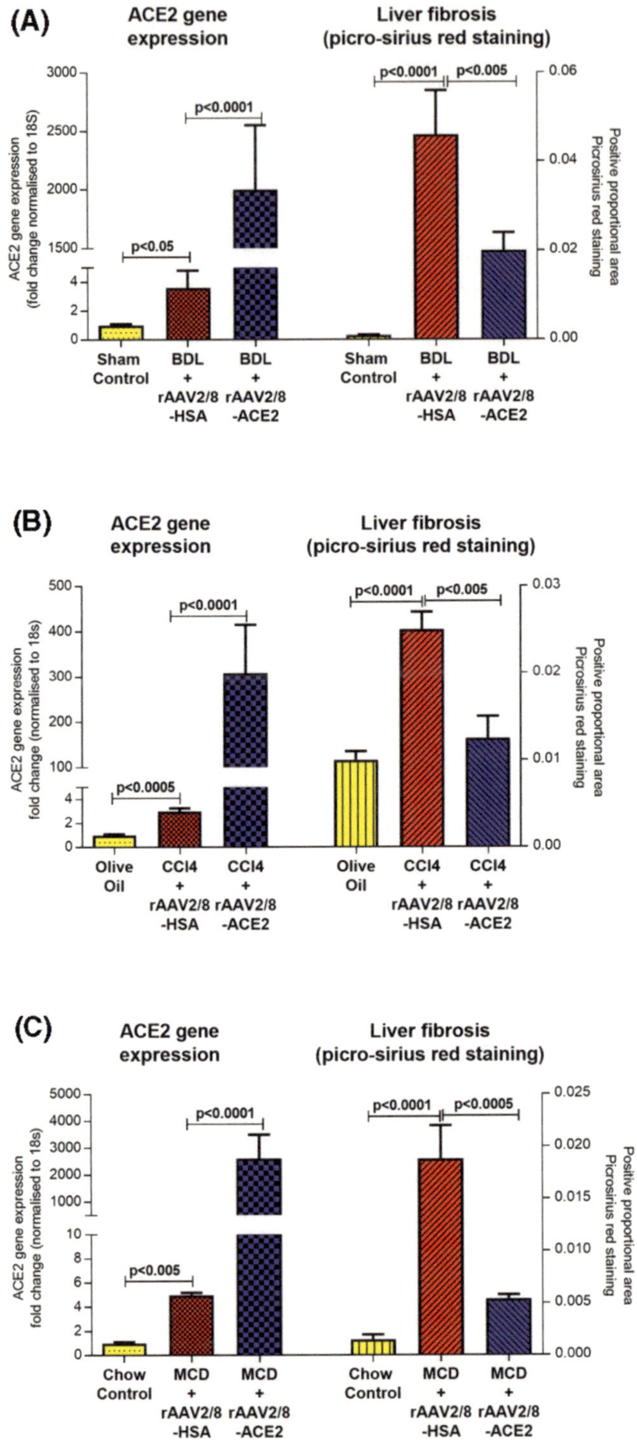

Figure 2. Hepatic ACE2 gene expression and fibrosis in three short-term models of liver fibrosis with rAAV2/8-ACE2 therapy. ACE2 gene expression (A–C) was significantly increased ($p < 0.0001$) in ACE2-treated diseased mice compared to control vector (rAAV2/8-HSA) injected diseased mice of BDL, CCl4, and MCD. As a result, rAAV2/8-ACE2 gene therapy has markedly reduced the liver fibrosis in each mouse model (BDL, CCl4, and MCD).

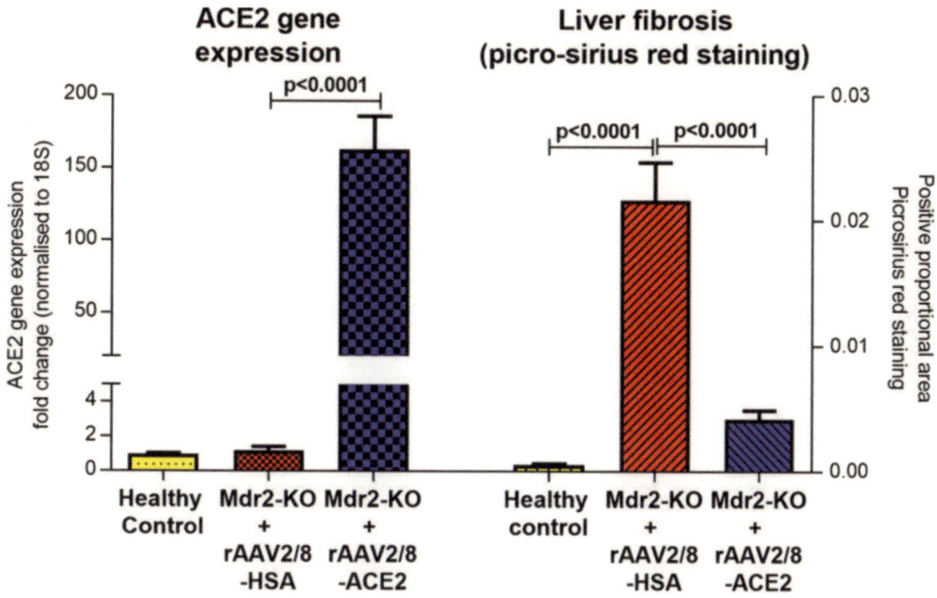

Figure 3. rAAV2/8-ACE2 therapy in Mdr2-KO mice with hepatic fibrosis. rAAV2/8-ACE2 gene therapy has markedly increased the ACE2 gene expression in Mdr2-KO mice, whereas liver fibrosis was significantly reduced by the therapy in ACE2-treated mice compared to the control vector-injected Mdr2-KO mice.

AAV vectors [93], we found that rAAV2/8-ACE2 reduced serum alanine transaminase (ALT) levels in diseased animals compared to those that received the control vector (rAAV2/8-HSA), suggesting that the vector itself is safe in the liver. Moreover, rAAV2/8-HSA (up to 10 days) or rAAV2/8-ACE2 (up to 24 weeks) vector injected into healthy mice produced no change in plasma ALT level, confirming that the vector itself is unlikely to cause liver injury [6, 87]. The schematic representation of molecular mechanism associated with ACE2 gene therapy using rAAV2/8 vector in hepatic fibrosis is shown in **Figure 4**.

Liver-targeted gene delivery using rAAV2/8 vector has shown to be therapeutically promising in adult liver, but their effects have not been extensively investigated in the immature liver. Although rAAV2/8 transduces neonatal mouse liver with high efficiency, the vector is not persistent in the liver and declines rapidly with liver growth [127]. Therefore, the successful use of rAAV2/8-mediated therapy to treat liver disease in early childhood may require readministration [128]. In line with this, another study demonstrated that the treatment of ornithine transcarbamylase (OTC)-deficient neonatal mice with AAV2/8-OTC therapy failed to protect mice from hyperammonemia in adulthood [129]. Thus, producing stable transduction in the developing liver remains one of the biggest challenges for liver-specific rAAV2/8 gene therapy, and readministration of vectors may be necessary to maintain therapeutic efficacy in adulthood after early neonatal treatment.

Although the AAV vectors employed for preclinical studies may be effective in human liver, it is important to select an AAV vector specific for human hepatocytes with enhanced transduction efficiency [6, 55]. Recently, two groups have proposed using humanized mice such as the immunosuppressed FRG ($Fah^{-/-}/Rag2^{-/-}/Il2rg^{-/-}$) mouse model to identify the best rAAV serotype for liver-directed gene therapy [55, 130]. The studies in humanized

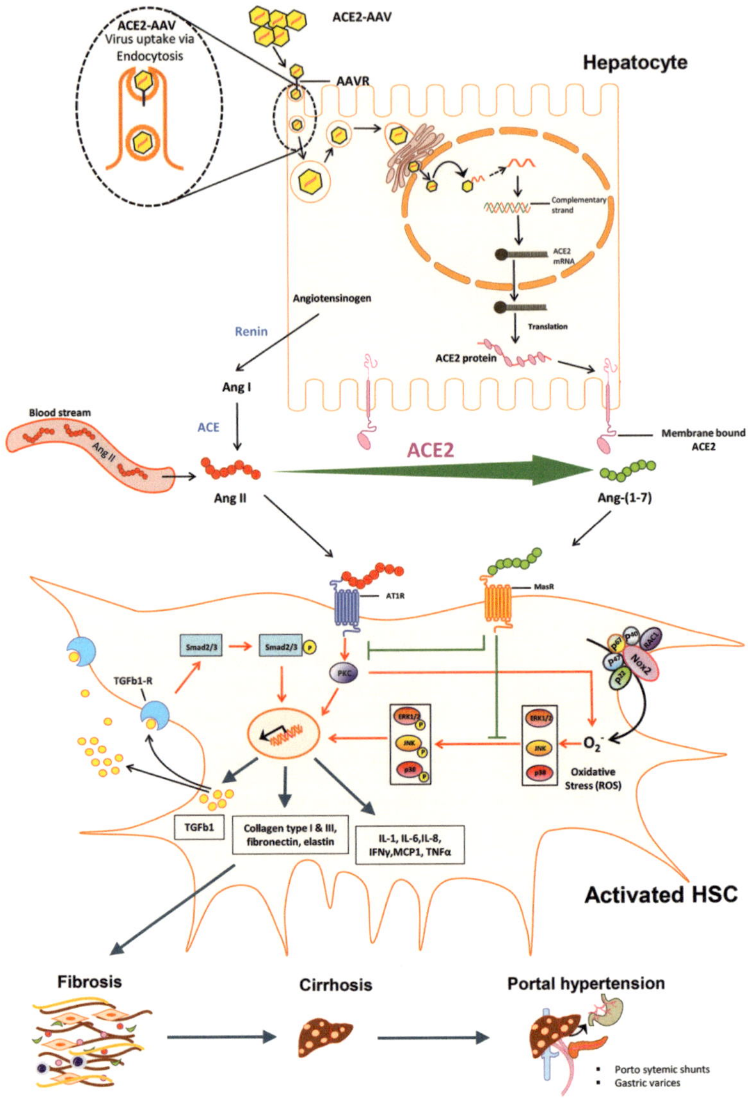

Figure 4. rAAV2/8-ACE2 uptake by hepatocytes and a cascade of events triggered by ACE2 protein in activated hepatic stellate cells (HSCs) during fibrosis. rAAV-ACE2 particles use AAV receptor (AAV-R) on hepatocyte membrane to enter the cytoplasm, followed by translocation into nucleus where uncoating and releasing of single-stranded viral genome occurs. The complementary strand will then be synthesized to transcribe ACE2. Membrane bound ACE2 protein has an exclusive role of cleaving potent profibrotic peptide angiotensin II (Ang II) to antifibrotic peptide angiotensin-1-7 (Ang-(1–7)). While a reduction in local Ang II levels leads to a significant reduction in the activation of its receptor, Ang II type 1 (AT1-R), Ang-(1–7) working through its receptor, Mas (Mas-R), inhibits the AT1-R activated downstream signaling such as PKC- and NADPH-mediated ROS production in activated HSCs. This in turn inhibits the phosphorylation of MAPKs such as ERK1/2, JNK, and p38, leading to a reduction in proinflammatory cytokines such as IL-1, IL-6, IL-8, IFNγ, MCP-1, and TNFα and profibrotic cytokine TGFβ1. A reduction in the activity of TGFβ1 leads to a reduction in phosphorylation of its transcription factors, Smad2/3, resulting in the inhibition of secretion of matrix proteins such as collagens and fibronectins. Thus, rAAV-ACE2 helps improving hepatic fibrosis and thus, intrahepatic vascular tone, leading to an improvement in portal hypertension. PKC, protein kinase C; NADPH oxidase, nicotinamide adenine dinucleotide phosphate oxidase; IL, interleukin; IFNγ, interferon γ; MCP-1, monocyte chemotactic protein 1; TNFα, tumor necrosis factor α; TGFβ1, transforming growth factor-β1; ERK1/2, extracellular regulated kinase1/2; JNK, C-Jun N-terminal kinase.

http://dx.doi.org/10.5772/intechopen.80317

mouse model repopulated with over 25% human hepatocytes allowed the researchers to identify human liver-specific AAV vectors such as LK-03 derived from capsid DNA-shuffled AAV library. This library was generated using 10 AAV capsid genes. LK-03, which is composed of five different parental AAV capsids, was able to transduce human primary hepatocytes at higher efficiency *in vitro* and in a hepatocellular carcinoma xenograft model *in vivo* when compared to AAV serotype 8 [55]. Wang and colleagues also reported a higher liver transduction level in FRG mice using capsid of AAVrh10, a clade E AAV derived from rhesus macaque, and AAV3B and have shown that AAV-LK-03 vectors may be superior to either AAV3B or AAV8 [131]. It is expected that researchers will increasingly use humanized animal models for diseases other than liver disease, which will allow them to identify novel variants of engineered AAV vectors, transduction efficiency, and immune reactions specific to the human tissue under investigation. Moreover, it has been reported that AAV3B-eGFP vector, which was able to cause liver-specific robust GFP expression in the livers of non-human primates, is significantly better than AAV8 with no apparent hepatotoxicity [132].

13. Conclusions

Much of preclinical studies which employed a diverse range of naturally occurring as well as engineered AAV vectors in the last decade provided ample evidence that therapeutic gene transfer certainly holds a great promise for patients with inherited disorders such as those that developed as a result of blood clotting factor deficiency and mutated retinal genes causing blindness. Moreover, it is now becoming clear that the findings of preclinical studies of non-inherited disorders suggest that clinical studies utilizing therapeutic gene transfer is feasible.

Currently active clinical trials in patients with inherited disorders using a diverse range of AAV vector types will be expected to provide valuable insights into the safety and efficacy of AAV vectors [133]. Since the FDA as well as the EU has now endorsed human gene therapy, there is every possibility that the volume of gene therapy research employing next-generation AAV vectors for both inherited and non-inherited disorders in both preclinical and clinical settings would be expected to increase in the coming years. Moreover, a rapidly evolving technology of AAV vector engineering and the use of humanized animal models would be a key for rapid translation of preclinical findings to clinical studies. The findings from our ongoing liver fibrosis/cirrhosis work using human liver-specific AAV-LK-03 vector in humanized FRG mice would be expected to provide valuable information before we commence clinical studies in patients with chronic liver disease.

Author details

Indu Rajapaksha, Peter Angus and Chandana Herath*

*Address all correspondence to: cherath@unimelb.edu.au

The University of Melbourne, Melbourne, Australia

References

[1] Atchison RW, Casto BC, Hammon WM. Adenovirus-associated defective virus particles. Science. 1965;**149**:754-755

[2] Carter BJ. Adeno-associated virus and the development of adeno-associated virus vectors: A historical perspective. Molecular Therapy. 2004;**10**:981-989

[3] Srivastava A, Lusby EW, Berns KI. Nucleotide sequence and organization of the adeno-associated virus 2 genome. Journal of Virology. 1983;**45**:555-564

[4] Hildinger M, Auricchio A. Advances in AAV-mediated gene transfer for the treatment of inherited disorders. European Journal of Human Genetics. 2004;**12**:263

[5] Hoggan MD. Adenovirus associated viruses. Progress in Medical Virology. Fortschritte der medizinischen Virusforschung. Progres en Virologie Medicale. 1970;**12**:211-239

[6] Kai YM, Indu GR, Peter WA, Chandana BH. The adeno-associated virus—A safe and promising vehicle for liverspecific gene therapy of inherited and non-inherited disorders. Current Gene Therapy. 2017;**17**:4-16

[7] De La Maza LM, Carter BJ. Molecular structure of adeno-associated virus variant DNA. Journal of Biological Chemistry. 1980;**255**:3194-3203

[8] Lusby E, Fife KH, Berns KI. Nucleotide sequence of the inverted terminal repetition in adeno-associated virus DNA. Journal of Virology. 1980;**34**:402-409

[9] Xie Q et al. The atomic structure of adeno-associated virus (AAV-2), a vector for human gene therapy. Proceedings of the National Academy of Sciences. 2002;**99**:10405

[10] Hermonat PL, Labow MA, Wright R, Berns KI, Muzyczka N. Genetics of adeno-associated virus: Isolation and preliminary characterization of adeno-associated virus type 2 mutants. Journal of Virology. 1984;**51**:329-339

[11] Wu P et al. Mutational analysis of the adeno-associated virus type 2 (AAV2) capsid gene and construction of AAV2 vectors with altered tropism. Journal of Virology. 2000; **74**:8635-8647

[12] Hoque M et al. Nuclear transport of the major capsid protein is essential for adeno- associated virus capsid formation. Journal of Virology. 1999;**73**:7912-7915

[13] Summerford C, Samulski RJ. Membrane-associated heparan sulfate proteoglycan is a receptor for adeno-associated virus type 2 virions. Journal of Virology. 1998;**72**:1438-1445

[14] Rabinowitz JE, Xiao W, Samulski RJ. Insertional mutagenesis of AAV2 capsid and the production of recombinant virus. Virology. 1999;**265**:274-285

[15] Summerford C, Bartlett JS, Samulski RJ. $\alpha V\beta 5$ integrin: A co-receptor for adeno-associated virus type 2 infection. Nature Medicine. 1999;**5**:78

[16] Qing K et al. Human fibroblast growth factor receptor 1 is a co-receptor for infection by adeno-associated virus 2. Nature Medicine. 1999;**5**:71

[17] Handa A, Muramatsu SI, Qiu J, Mizukami H, Brown KE. Adeno-associated virus (AAV)-3-based vectors transduce haematopoietic cells not susceptible to transduction with AAV-2-based vectors. Journal of General Virology. 2000;**81**:2077-2084

[18] Schmidt M et al. Molecular characterization of the heparin-dependent transduction domain on the capsid of a novel adeno-associated virus isolate, AAV(VR-942). Journal of Virology. 2008;**82**:8911-8916

[19] Kaludov N, Brown KE, Walters RW, Zabner J, Chiorini JA. Adeno-associated virus serotype 4 (AAV4) and AAV5 both require sialic acid binding for hemagglutination and efficient transduction but differ in sialic acid linkage specificity. Journal of Virology. 2001;**75**:6884-6893

[20] Wu Z, Miller E, Agbandje-McKenna M, Samulski RJ. α2,3 and α2,6 N-linked sialic acids facilitate efficient binding and transduction by adeno-associated virus types 1 and 6. Journal of Virology. 2006;**80**:9093-9103

[21] Shen S, Bryant KD, Brown SM, Randell SH, Asokan A. Terminal N-linked galactose is the primary receptor for adeno-associated virus 9. The Journal of Biological Chemistry. 2011;**286**:13532-13540

[22] Asokan A, Hamra JB, Govindasamy L, Agbandje-McKenna M, Samulski RJ. Adeno-associated virus type 2 contains an integrin $\alpha 5\beta 1$ binding domain essential for viral cell entry. Journal of Virology. 2006;**80**:8961-8969

[23] Kashiwakura Y et al. Hepatocyte growth factor receptor is a coreceptor for adeno-associated virus type 2 infection. Journal of Virology. 2005;**79**:609-614

[24] Akache B et al. The 37/67-kilodalton laminin receptor is a receptor for adeno-associated virus serotypes 8, 2, 3, and 9. Journal of Virology. 2006;**80**:9831-9836

[25] Pillay S et al. An essential receptor for adeno-associated virus infection. Nature. 2016; **530**:108-112

[26] Sanlioglu S et al. Endocytosis and nuclear trafficking of adeno-associated virus type 2 are controlled by Rac1 and phosphatidylinositol-3 kinase activation. Journal of Virology. 2000;**74**:9184-9196

[27] Ren C, White AF, Ponnazhagan S. Notch1 augments intracellular trafficking of adeno-associated virus type 2. Journal of Virology. 2007;**81**:2069-2073

[28] Sonntag F, Bleker S, Leuchs B, Fischer R, Kleinschmidt JA. Adeno-associated virus type 2 capsids with externalized VP1/VP2 trafficking domains are generated prior to passage through the cytoplasm and are maintained until uncoating occurs in the nucleus. Journal of Virology. 2006;**80**:11040-11054

[29] Douar A-M, Poulard K, Stockholm D, Danos O. Intracellular trafficking of adeno-associated virus vectors: Routing to the late endosomal compartment and proteasome degradation. Journal of Virology. 2001;**75**:1824-1833

[30] Hansen J, Qing K, Srivastava A. Adeno-associated virus type 2-mediated gene transfer: Altered endocytic processing enhances transduction efficiency in murine fibroblasts. Journal of Virology. 2001;**75**:4080-4090

[31] Pajusola K et al. Cell-type-specific characteristics modulate the transduction efficiency of adeno-associated virus type 2 and restrain infection of endothelial cells. Journal of Virology. 2002;**76**:11530-11540

[32] Yan Z et al. Distinct classes of proteasome-modulating agents cooperatively augment recombinant adeno-associated virus type 2 and type 5-mediated transduction from the apical surfaces of human airway epithelia. Journal of Virology. 2004;**78**:2863-2874

[33] Duan D, Yue Y, Yan Z, Yang J, Engelhardt JF. Endosomal processing limits gene transfer to polarized airway epithelia by adeno-associated virus. Journal of Clinical Investigation. 2000;**105**:1573-1587

[34] Girod A et al. The VP1 capsid protein of adeno-associated virus type 2 is carrying a phospholipase A2 domain required for virus infectivity. Journal of General Virology. 2002;**83**:973-978

[35] Xiao PJ, Li C, Neumann A, Samulski RJ. Quantitative 3D tracing of gene-delivery viral vectors in human cells and animal tissues. Molecular Therapy. 2012;**20**:317-328

[36] Li C et al. Adeno-associated virus capsid antigen presentation is dependent on endosomal escape. The Journal of Clinical Investigation. 2013;**123**:1390-1401

[37] Nicolson SC, Samulski RJ. Recombinant adeno-associated virus utilizes host cell nuclear import machinery to enter the nucleus. Journal of Virology. 2014;**88**:4132-4144

[38] Kann M, Sodeik B, Vlachou A, Gerlich WH, Helenius A. Phosphorylation-dependent binding of hepatitis B virus core particles to the nuclear pore complex. The Journal of Cell Biology. 1999;**145**:45-55

[39] Ojala PM, Sodeik B, Ebersold MW, Kutay U, Helenius A. Herpes simplex virus type 1 entry into host cells: Reconstitution of capsid binding and uncoating at the nuclear pore complex in vitro. Molecular and Cellular Biology. 2000;**20**:4922-4931

[40] Kelich JM et al. Super-resolution imaging of nuclear import of adeno-associated virus in live cells. Molecular Therapy. Methods and Clinical Development. 2015;**2**:15047

[41] Qiu J, Brown KE. A 110-kDa nuclear shuttle protein, nucleolin, specifically binds to adeno-associated virus type 2 (AAV-2) capsid. Virology. 1999;**257**:373-382

[42] Gonçalves MA. Adeno-associated virus: From defective virus to effective vector. Virology Journal. 2005;**2**:43

[43] McCarty DM. Self-complementary AAV vectors; Advances and applications. Molecular Therapy. 2008;**16**:1648-1656

[44] Gruenert AK et al. Self-complementary adeno-associated virus vectors improve transduction efficiency of corneal endothelial cells. PLoS One. 2016;**11**:e0152589

[45] Maina N et al. Recombinant self-complementary adeno-associated virus serotype vector-mediated hematopoietic stem cell transduction and lineage-restricted, long-term transgene expression in a murine serial bone marrow transplantation model. Human Gene Therapy. 2008;**19**:376-383

[46] Wang Z et al. Rapid and highly efficient transduction by double-stranded adeno-associated virus vectors in vitro and in vivo. Gene Therapy. 2003;**10**:2105

[47] Fu H et al. Self-complementary adeno-associated virus serotype 2 vector: Global distribution and broad dispersion of AAV-mediated transgene expression in mouse brain. Molecular Therapy. 2003;**8**:911-917

[48] Nathwani AC et al. Safe and efficient transduction of the liver after peripheral vein infusion of self-complementary AAV vector results in stable therapeutic expression of human FIX in nonhuman primates. Blood. 2007;**109**:1414-1421

[49] Natkunarajah M et al. Assessment of ocular transduction using single-stranded and self-complementary recombinant adeno-associated virus serotype 2/8. Gene Therapy. 2007;**15**:463

[50] Vance MA, Mitchell A, Samulski RJ. AAV biology, infectivity and therapeutic use from bench to clinic. In: Hashad D, editor. Gene Therapy—Principles and Challenges. Ch. 05. Rijeka: InTech; 2015

[51] Gao G et al. Adeno-associated viruses undergo substantial evolution in primates during natural infections. Proceedings of the National Academy of Sciences of the United States of America. 2003;**100**:6081-6086

[52] Zincarelli C, Soltys S, Rengo G, Rabinowitz JE. Analysis of AAV serotypes 1-9 mediated gene expression and tropism in mice after systemic injection. Molecular Therapy. 2008;**16**:1073-1080

[53] Nam H-J et al. Structure of adeno-associated virus serotype 8, a gene therapy vector. Journal of Virology. 2007;**81**:12260-12271

[54] Grimm D et al. In vitro and in vivo gene therapy vector evolution via multispecies interbreeding and retargeting of adeno-associated viruses. Journal of Virology. 2008; **82**:5887-5911

[55] Lisowski L et al. Selection and evaluation of clinically relevant AAV variants in a xenograft liver model. Nature. 2013;**506**:382

[56] Zinn E et al. In silico reconstruction of the viral evolutionary lineage yields a potent gene therapy vector. Cell Reports. 2015;**12**:1056-1068

[57] Vandendriessche T et al. Efficacy and safety of adeno-associated viral vectors based on serotype 8 and 9 vs. lentiviral vectors for hemophilia B gene therapy. Journal of Thrombosis and Haemostasis. 2007;**5**:16-24

[58] Zhu J, Huang X, Yang Y. The TLR9-MyD88 pathway is critical for adaptive immune responses to adeno-associated virus gene therapy vectors in mice. The Journal of Clinical Investigation. 2009;**119**:2388-2398

[59] Li Q et al. Intraocular route of AAV2 vector administration defines humoral immune response and therapeutic potential. Molecular Vision. 2008;**14**:1760-1769

[60] Halbert CL, Standaert TA, Wilson CB, Miller AD. Successful readministration of adeno-associated virus vectors to the mouse lung requires transient immunosuppression during the initial exposure. Journal of Virology. 1998;**72**:9795-9805

[61] Hildinger M et al. Hybrid vectors based on adeno-associated virus serotypes 2 and 5 for muscle-directed gene transfer. Journal of Virology. 2001;**75**:6199-6203

[62] Blacklow NR, Hoggan MD, Rowe WP. Serologic evidence for human infection with adenovirus-associated viruses. Journal of the National Cancer Institute. 1968;**40**:319-327

[63] Calcedo R et al. Adeno-associated virus antibody profiles in newborns, children, and adolescents. Clinical and Vaccine Immunology. 2011;**18**:1586-1588

[64] Calcedo R, Vandenberghe LH, Gao G, Lin J, Wilson JM. Worldwide epidemiology of neutralizing antibodies to adeno-associated viruses. The Journal of Infectious Diseases. 2009;**199**:381-390

[65] Xin K-Q et al. Induction of robust immune responses against human immunodeficiency virus is supported by the inherent tropism of adeno-associated virus type 5 for dendritic cells. Journal of Virology. 2006;**80**:11899-11910

[66] Veron P et al. Major subsets of human dendritic cells are efficiently transduced by self-complementary adeno-associated virus vectors 1 and 2. Journal of Virology. 2007;**81**:5385-5394

[67] Lu Y, Song S. Distinct immune responses to transgene products from rAAV1 and rAAV8 vectors. Proceedings of the National Academy of Sciences of the United States of America. 2009;**106**:17158-17162

[68] Maguire CA et al. Mouse gender influences brain transduction by intravascularly administered AAV9. Molecular Therapy. 2013;**21**:1470-1471

[69] Davidoff AM, Ng CYC, Zhou J, Spence Y, Nathwani AC. Sex significantly influences transduction of murine liver by recombinant adeno-associated viral vectors through an androgen-dependent pathway. Blood. 2003;**102**:480

[70] Dane AP, Cunningham SC, Graf NS, Alexander IE. Sexually dimorphic patterns of episomal rAAV genome persistence in the adult mouse liver and correlation with hepatocellular proliferation. Molecular Therapy: The Journal of the American Society of Gene Therapy. 2009;**17**:1548-1554

[71] Kaplitt MG et al. Long-term gene expression and phenotypic correction using adeno-associated virus vectors in the mammalian brain. Nature Genetics. 1994;**8**:148

[72] Flannery JG et al. Efficient photoreceptor-targeted gene expression in vivo by recombinant adeno-associated virus. Proceedings of the National Academy of Sciences of the United States of America. 1997;**94**:6916-6921

[73] Fisher KJ et al. Recombinant adeno-associated virus for muscle directed gene therapy. Nature Medicine. 1997;**3**:306

[74] Snyder RO et al. Persistent and therapeutic concentrations of human factor IX in mice after hepatic gene transfer of recombinant AAV vectors. Nature Genetics. 1997;**16**:270

[75] Xiao W et al. Adeno-associated virus as a vector for liver-directed gene therapy. Journal of Virology. 1998;**72**:10222-10226

[76] Snyder RO et al. Correction of hemophilia B in canine and murine models using recombinant adeno-associated viral vectors. Nature Medicine. 1999;**5**:64

[77] Guangping G, Luk HV, James MW. New recombinant serotypes of AAV vectors. Current Gene Therapy. 2005;**5**:285-297

[78] Health, T.U.N.I.o. The US National Institute of Health. Adeno-associated virus. 2016. Available from: https://clinicaltrials.gov/ct2/results?term=adeno+associated+virus&Search=Search

[79] Gao G-P et al. Novel adeno-associated viruses from rhesus monkeys as vectors for human gene therapy. Proceedings of the National Academy of Sciences of the United States of America. 2002;**99**:11854-11859

[80] Nakai H et al. Unrestricted hepatocyte transduction with adeno-associated virus serotype 8 vectors in mice. Journal of Virology. 2005;**79**:214-224

[81] Nathwani AC et al. Self-complementary adeno-associated virus vectors containing a novel liver-specific human factor IX expression cassette enable highly efficient transduction of murine and nonhuman primate liver. Blood. 2006;**107**:2653-2661

[82] McCarty DM et al. Adeno-associated virus terminal repeat (TR) mutant generates self-complementary vectors to overcome the rate-limiting step to transduction in vivo. Gene Therapy. 2003;**10**:2112

[83] Matsushita T et al. Adeno-associated virus vectors can be efficiently produced without helper virus. Gene Therapy. 1998;**5**:938

[84] Xiao X, Li J, Samulski RJ. Production of high-titer recombinant adeno-associated virus vectors in the absence of helper adenovirus. Journal of Virology. 1998;**72**:2224-2232

[85] McClure C, Cole KLH, Wulff P, Klugmann M, Murray AJ. Production and titering of recombinant adeno-associated viral vectors. Journal of Visualized Experiments. 2011;JoVE(57):e3348. DOI: 10.3791/3348

[86] Grieger JC, Choi VW, Samulski RJ. Production and characterization of adeno-associated viral vectors. Nature Protocols. 2006;**1**:1412

[87] Mak KY et al. ACE2 therapy using adeno-associated viral vector inhibits liver fibrosis in mice. Molecular Therapy. 2015;**23**:1434-1443

[88] Allen NA, Samulski RJ. The pros and cons of using the mechanism of AAV site-specific recombination in gene delivery. Gene Therapy and Regulation. 2004;**2**:121-138

[89] Monahan PE, Samulski RJ. Adeno-associated virus vectors for gene therapy: More pros than cons? Molecular Medicine Today. 2000;**6**:433-440

[90] Ferreira V, Petry H, Salmon F. Immune responses to AAV-vectors, the glybera example from bench to bedside. Frontiers in Immunology. 2014;**5**:82

[91] Senior M. After Glybera's withdrawal, what's next for gene therapy? Nature Biotechnology. 2017;**35**:491

[92] Ursula K, Tim H, Thomas G, Marion WD, Bastian S, Ilja D, Elisabeth ST, et al. Gene therapy in lipoprotein lipase deficiency (LPLD): Case report on the first patient treated with alipogene tiparvovec under daily practice conditions. Human Gene Therapy. 2018;**29**(4):520-527. DOI: 10.1089/hum.2018.007

[93] Nathwani AC et al. Long-term safety and efficacy of factor IX gene therapy in hemophilia B. New England Journal of Medicine. 2014;**371**:1994-2004

[94] Herzog RW et al. Stable gene transfer and expression of human blood coagulation factor IX after intramuscular injection of recombinant adeno-associated virus. Proceedings of the National Academy of Sciences of the United States of America. 1997;**94**:5804-5809

[95] Wang L et al. Sustained correction of disease in naive and AAV2-pretreated hemophilia B dogs: AAV2/8-mediated, liver-directed gene therapy. Blood. 2005;**105**:3079-3086

[96] Herzog RW et al. Long-term correction of canine hemophilia B by gene transfer of blood coagulation factor IX mediated by adeno-associated viral vector. Nature Medicine. 1999;**5**:56

[97] Wang L, Nichols TC, Read MS, Bellinger DA, Verma IM. Sustained expression of therapeutic level of factor IX in hemophilia B dogs by AAV-mediated gene therapy in liver. Molecular Therapy. 2000;**1**:154-158

[98] Mingozzi F et al. Induction of immune tolerance to coagulation factor IX antigen by in vivo hepatic gene transfer. Journal of Clinical Investigation. 2003;**111**:1347-1356

[99] Manno CS et al. AAV-mediated factor IX gene transfer to skeletal muscle in patients with severe hemophilia B. Blood. 2003;**101**:2963-2972

[100] Manno CS et al. Successful transduction of liver in hemophilia by AAV-Factor IX and limitations imposed by the host immune response. Nature Medicine. 2006;**12**:342

[101] Nathwani AC et al. Adenovirus-associated virus vector–mediated gene transfer in hemophilia B. New England Journal of Medicine. 2011;**365**:2357-2365

[102] George LA et al. Hemophilia B gene therapy with a high-specific-activity factor IX variant. New England Journal of Medicine. 2017;**377**:2215-2227

[103] George LA. Hemophilia gene therapy comes of age. Blood Advances. 2017;**1**:2591-2599

[104] Bainbridge JWB et al. Effect of gene therapy on visual function in Leber's congenital amaurosis. New England Journal of Medicine. 2008;**358**:2231-2239

[105] Cai X, Conley SM, Naash MI. RPE65: Role in the visual cycle, human retinal disease, and gene therapy. Ophthalmic Genetics. 2009;**30**:57

[106] Hauswirth WW et al. Treatment of Leber congenital amaurosis due to RPE65 mutations by ocular subretinal injection of adeno-associated virus gene vector: Short-term results of a phase I trial. Human Gene Therapy. 2008;**19**:979-990

[107] Cideciyan AV et al. Human RPE65 gene therapy for Leber congenital amaurosis: Persistence of early visual improvements and safety at 1 year. Human Gene Therapy. 2009;**20**:999-1004

[108] Schuppan D, Kim YO. Evolving therapies for liver fibrosis. The Journal of Clinical Investigation. 2013;**123**:1887-1901

[109] Povedano JM et al. Therapeutic effects of telomerase in mice with pulmonary fibrosis induced by damage to the lungs and short telomeres. eLife. 2018;**7**:e31299

[110] Chamberlain KR, Jalish M, Weber T. Cardiac gene therapy with adeno-associated virus-based vectors. Current Opinion in Cardiology. 2017;**32**:275-282

[111] Jaski BE et al. Calcium upregulation by percutaneous administration of gene therapy in cardiac disease (CUPID Trial), a first-in-human phase 1/2 clinical trial. Circulation. 2011;**124**:304-313

[112] Zsebo K et al. Long-term effects of AAV1/SERCA2a gene transfer in patients with severe heart failure-novelty and significance. Analysis of Recurrent Cardiovascular Events and Mortality. 2014;**114**:101-108

[113] Greenberg B et al. Design of a phase 2b trial of intracoronary administration of AAV1/SERCA2a in patients with advanced heart failure: The CUPID 2 trial (calcium up-regulation by percutaneous administration of gene therapy in cardiac disease phase 2b). JACC: Heart Failure. 2014;**2**:84-92

[114] Asokan A et al. Reengineering a receptor footprint of adeno-associated virus enables selective and systemic gene transfer to muscle. Nature Biotechnology. 2010;**28**:79-82

[115] Ishikawa K et al. Cardiac I-1c overexpression with reengineered AAV improves cardiac function in swine ischemic heart failure. Molecular Therapy. 2014;**22**:2038-2045

[116] Hocquemiller M, Giersch L, Audrain M, Parker S, Cartier N. Adeno-associated virus-based gene therapy for CNS diseases. Human Gene Therapy. 2016;**27**:478-496

[117] Fischer G, Pan B, Vilceanu D, Hogan QH, Yu H. Sustained relief of neuropathic pain by AAV-targeted expression of CBD3 peptide in rat dorsal root ganglion. Gene Therapy. 2014;**21**:44-51

[118] Hirai T et al. Intrathecal AAV serotype 9-mediated delivery of shRNA against TRPV1 attenuates thermal hyperalgesia in a mouse model of peripheral nerve injury. Molecular Therapy. 2014;**22**:409-419

[119] Tandon P, Abraldes JG, Berzigotti A, Garcia-Pagan JC, Bosch J. Renin angiotensin-aldosterone inhibitors in the reduction of portal pressure: A systematic review and meta-analysis. Journal of Hepatology. 2010;**53**:273-282

[120] Herath CB et al. Upregulation of hepatic angiotensin-converting enzyme 2 (ACE2) and angiotensin-(1-7) levels in experimental biliary fibrosis. Journal of Hepatology. 2007; **47**:387-395

[121] Paizis G et al. Chronic liver injury in rats and humans upregulates the novel enzyme angiotensin converting enzyme 2. Gut. 2005;**54**:1790-1796

[122] Wysocki J et al. Targeting the degradation of angiotensin II with recombinant angiotensin-converting enzyme 2. Hypertension. 2009;**55**:90

[123] Oudit GY et al. Human recombinant ACE2 reduces the progression of diabetic nephropathy. Diabetes. 2010;**59**:529

[124] Haschke M et al. Pharmacokinetics and pharmacodynamics of recombinant human angiotensin-converting enzyme 2 in healthy human subjects. Clinical Pharmacokinetics. 2013;**52**:783-792

[125] Österreicher CH et al. Angiotensin-converting-enzyme 2 inhibits liver fibrosis in mice. Hepatology (Baltimore, Md.). 2009;**50**:929-938

[126] Herath CB, Mak KY, Angus PW. Chapter 34 - Role of the alternate RAS in liver disease and the GI tract. In: Unger T, Steckelings UM, dos Santos RAS, editors. The Protective Arm of the Renin Angiotensin System (RAS). Boston: Academic Press; 2015. pp. 239-247. doi.org/10.1016/B978-0-12-801364-9.00034-1

[127] Cunningham SC, Dane AP, Spinoulas A, Alexander IE. Gene delivery to the juvenile mouse liver using AAV2/8 vectors. Molecular Therapy. 2008;**16**:1081-1088

[128] Wang L, Wang H, Bell P, McMenamin D, Wilson JM. Hepatic gene transfer in neonatal mice by adeno-associated virus serotype 8 vector. Human Gene Therapy. 2012; **23**:533-539

[129] Cunningham SC, Kok CY, Spinoulas A, Carpenter KH, Alexander IE. AAV-encoded OTC activity persisting to adulthood following delivery to newborn spfash mice is insufficient to prevent shRNA-induced hyperammonaemia. Gene Therapy. 2013;**20**:1184

[130] Azuma H et al. Robust expansion of human hepatocytes in Fah(−/−)/Rag2(−/−)/Il2rg (−/−) mice. Nature Biotechnology. 2007;**25**:903-910

[131] Wang L et al. Comparative study of liver gene transfer with AAV vectors based on natural and engineered AAV capsids. Molecular Therapy. 2015;**23**:1877-1887

[132] Li S et al. Efficient and targeted transduction of nonhuman primate liver with systemically delivered optimized AAV3B vectors. Molecular Therapy. 2015;**23**:1867-1876

[133] The US National Institute of Health. Adeno-associated virus. Available from: https://clinicaltrials.gov/ct2/results?term=adeno+associated

[134] Davidson BL et al. Recombinant adeno-associated virus type 2, 4, and 5 vectors: Transduction of variant cell types and regions in the mammalian central nervous system. Proceedings of the National Academy of Sciences of the United States of America. 2000;**97**:3428-3432

[135] Mori S, Wang L, Takeuchi T, Kanda T. Two novel adeno-associated viruses from cynomolgus monkey: Pseudotyping characterization of capsid protein. Virology. 2004; **330**:375-383

[136] Schmidt M et al. Adeno-associated virus type 12 (AAV12): A novel AAV serotype with sialic acid- and heparan sulfate proteoglycan-independent transduction activity. Journal of Virology. 2008;**82**:1399-1406

Section 3

Cardiac Gene Therapy

Chapter 8

Gene Therapy for Cardiomyopathies

Yves Fromes and Caroline Roques

Additional information is available at the end of the chapter

http://dx.doi.org/10.5772/intechopen.80478

Abstract

Heart disease remains the prevalent cause of premature death and accounts for a significant proportion of all hospital admissions. Molecular genetics was integrated quite late in cardiology, but introduced new concepts like sarcolemmopathies, cytoskeletalopathies, and channelopathies useful to better understand the pathophysiology of the development of inherited cardiomyopathies (CMs). As our understanding of the cellular and molecular processes involved in the development and progression of heart disease improved, new therapeutic targets were identified, as were novel approaches such as delivery of genes to replace defective or deficient components and thereby restore structure or function in a diseased heart. We discuss gene addition strategies in the context of monogenic disorders. Moreover, a broader nucleic acid-based modulation of cardiac gene expression for the treatment of cardiac diseases might have larger clinical indications. Inadequate gene delivery remains a potential cause of negative trials. However, progress in innovative formulations and clinically relevant ways of administration should lead to significant progress in the future. Cardiac gene therapy will be integrated into the therapeutic armamentarium for CM and heart failure.

Keywords: cardiomyopathy, heart failure, genetic disease, gene therapy, cardiac structure, cardiac function, viral vector, nanoparticles, polymers

1. Introduction: cardiomyopathies

Cardiomyopathies (CMs) refer basically to diseases of the heart muscle, which can be acquired or inherited [1]. CMs can affect people of all ages. However, people in certain age groups are more likely to have certain types of CMs, as inherited forms predominate in younger individuals and acquired diseases increase with age [2–8].

Most frequently, four main clinical forms are described, meaning hypertrophic, dilated, and restrictive types as well as arrhythmogenic CM. These diseases have many causes, signs, symptoms, and treatments. We exclude ischemic cardiopathies from this overview, and focus more precisely on disorders of the heart muscle of non-ischemic origin. This does, however, not exclude anomalies of the perfusion of the myocardium, because pathophysiology of these diseases is usually complex, interleaving different mechanisms.

Diagnosis of non-ischemic CM is a challenging process that influences patient morbidity and mortality. Multiple biomarkers and imaging tools contribute to the adequate ranking of the clinical presentation of these diseases. More recently, nuclear magnetic resonance (NMR) imaging appeared as a robust diagnostic tool that offers various techniques to assess the structure, function, perfusion, and scarring of myocardial tissue, thus providing better understanding of the underlying causes of CMs [9–12]. At a molecular level, genotyping identifies precisely the causal mutations in inherited forms of CMs. Moreover, a systems biology approach can investigate more fully the molecular profiles of different phenotypic stages of CM.

From a pathophysiological and diagnostic perspective, it might be useful to consider a stratification of CMs slightly different from the clinical classification. Considering the various genes that can trigger the development and evolution of a CM, we propose to group inherited diseases as cytoskeletal CMs or cytoskeletalopathies, sarcomeric CMs or sarcomyopathies, and finally ion channel CMs or channelopathies.

Different structural alterations of the myocardium contribute in varying degrees to the different forms of the diseases, but common features may represent as many therapeutic targets.

The focus of more extensive cellular degeneration is one of the histological hallmarks of CM [13,14]. Necrosis is not the only mechanism leading to cell death. Apoptosis, or programmed cell death, is a highly regulated and active process that contributes to the maintenance of adult cardiac tissue [15]. Myocyte cell death is implicated in the architectural rearrangement occurring in the surviving myocardium. This remodelling leads to heterogeneity in the myocardial structure, created by the altered behaviour of non-myocyte cells, particularly cardiac fibroblasts, which are responsible for myocardial collagen metabolism and fibrous tissue accumulation. It may largely explain the appearance of diastolic and/or systolic myocardial failure [15]. Adverse left ventricular remodelling leads to alteration in the structure (dimension, mass, shape) of the heart that might at the beginning of the process be considered as compensatory for the disease process, but at the end will severely impair cardiac function. Remodelling is also a prominent feature of electrophysiological properties of the myocardium, translated as clinical presentation such as atrial fibrillation, flutter, complete heart block, ventricular ectopic pacing, and tachycardia.

Considering the remodelling process as a deleterious end effect, one can raise the question of potential reverse remodelling. Could that be an option for remission or cure of CM? It has been shown that prolonged mechanical unloading of failing hearts can preserve myocardial contractility but impairs relaxation. Could gene therapy provide new therapeutic options for those patients?

Myocardial remodelling involves not only the cardiomyocytes, but also non-myocyte cells and the extracellular matrix. Fibrosis is an essential process in the repair of damaged tissues and wounds, but its accumulation in organs and tissues can lead to scarring, organ dysfunction, and, ultimately, failure. Development of interstitial and perivascular fibrosis of varying degrees is observed in most CMs. However, *in vivo* diagnosis of the extent and distribution of fibrosis remains difficult. New approaches such as ultrasound elastographic and cardiac NMR techniques might provide appropriate outcome measures to monitor more specifically myocardial fibrosis, and thus potential therapeutic effects [16].

Immune mechanisms modulate interstitial fibrosis, cardiomyocyte cell death, and hypertrophy, all of which are central processes leading to maladaptive remodelling in response to a variety of stimuli. Acute inflammation, as observed in myocarditis, might be out of the scope of the present overview, and would need a dedicated review. However, in chronic heart failure (CHF) patients, a chronic inflammatory activation has long been recognized. Heart failure is associated with a wide array of mechanisms subsumed under the term "inflammation." This chronic inflammation harms the myocardium instead of healing it. Gene therapy might find new therapeutic targets in this context.

Similarly to the structural modifications of the myocardium, functional alterations contribute to the definition of CM. From a perspective of pathophysiology, alterations of preload and afterload largely contribute to diastolic/systolic dysfunctions. Pressure–volume relationship best defines myocardium alteration beyond the hemodynamic parameters.

Moreover, a more detailed understanding of excitation–contraction coupling reveals new targets for innovative therapeutic strategies.

Furthermore, and beyond the triggering causes of CM, as heart muscle becomes weaker over time, a common clinical condition described as heart failure develops. From a pathophysiological and therapeutic perspective, heart failure could be considered as a specific disease stage, independent of the acquired or inherited origin of CM. Gene therapy could also be considered at this stage.

2. Therapeutic options: why gene therapy?

Many medicines are used to treat CM and CHF, but despite this, CM and CHF remain leading causes of morbidity and mortality even in developed countries. Correcting hemodynamic imbalances, such as fluid control (preload) or vascular resistance control (afterload), remains primordial, but cannot change the myocardial contractility *per se* (**Figure 1**). Fundamentally, determinants of cardiac output are the same as those of myocardial energy consumption. Therefore, tackling the problem of decreased contractility raises in parallel the problem of increased energy requirements. Several attempts to increase inotropism on a chronic basis led to overall negative results because energy consumption exceeded production. Gene therapy might offer new therapeutic options. The pressure–volume relationship demonstrates the contracting and relaxing portions of the cardiac cycle (**Figure 2**). The slope of the end-systolic

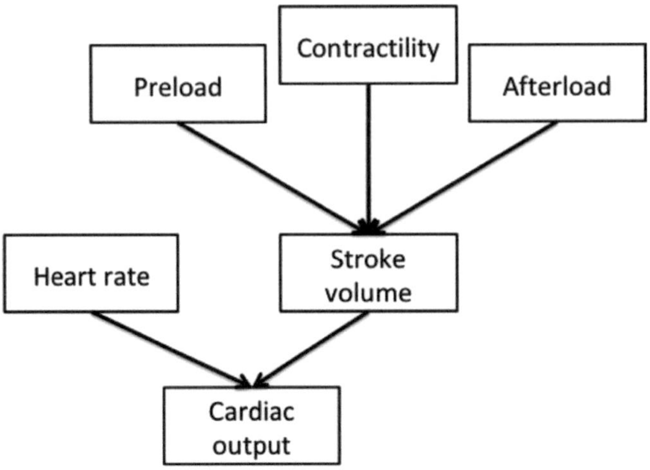

Figure 1. Determinants of cardiac output (CO). CO is the resultant of stroke volume, the difference between end-diastolic and end-systolic volumes times the heart rate. According to the Frank–Starling law, preload influences CO positively. With developing heart failure, CO is negatively influenced by afterload. Contractility represents the primary inotropic capacity of the myocardium.

pressure–volume relationship represents the most objective measure of the intrinsic contractile capacity of the myocardium.

Similarly, management of CHF patients frequently takes advantage of rhythm control (pharmacologic or pacemakers/implantable cardioverter defibrillator). Gene therapy might represent a new way to address this topic by recreating new endogenous biological pacemakers rather than relying on electronic devices.

Recent clinical trials [17–19] have not only pinpointed the importance of inflammation but moreover the therapeutic potentialities of selectively targeting some cytokines. At a preclinical level, glycoprotein-130 (gp130) has been identified as a potential new target [20–22]. It is now established that with gp-130, the common receptor of IL-6 is elevated in patients with chronic heart failure. Hilfiker-Kleiner et al. have shown that mice carrying a cardio-specific mutation of gp-130 have a normal myocardial phenotype at baseline. However, induction of an experimental myocardial infaction leads to development of heart failure and increased mortality. Moreover, these observations were associated with increased expression of complement-activating mannose-binding lectin [23]. Thus, this animal model suggested a link between IL-6 and chronic myocardial injury induced by complement activation.

Cardiac myofibroblasts respond to a large number of proinflammatory cytokines (e.g. TNF-alpha, IL-1, IL-6, TGF-beta), vasoactive peptides (e.g. angiotensin II, endothelin-1, natriuretic peptides), and hormones (e.g. noradrenaline), the levels of which are increased in the remodelling heart. Reducing myocardial remodelling specifically via modulatory effects on cardiac fibroblasts might represent further new therapeutic targets.

Anticoagulants in the context of CHF are an important therapeutic class for those subgroups of patients at high risk for abnormal clotting. Anticoagulation might appear inappropriate for

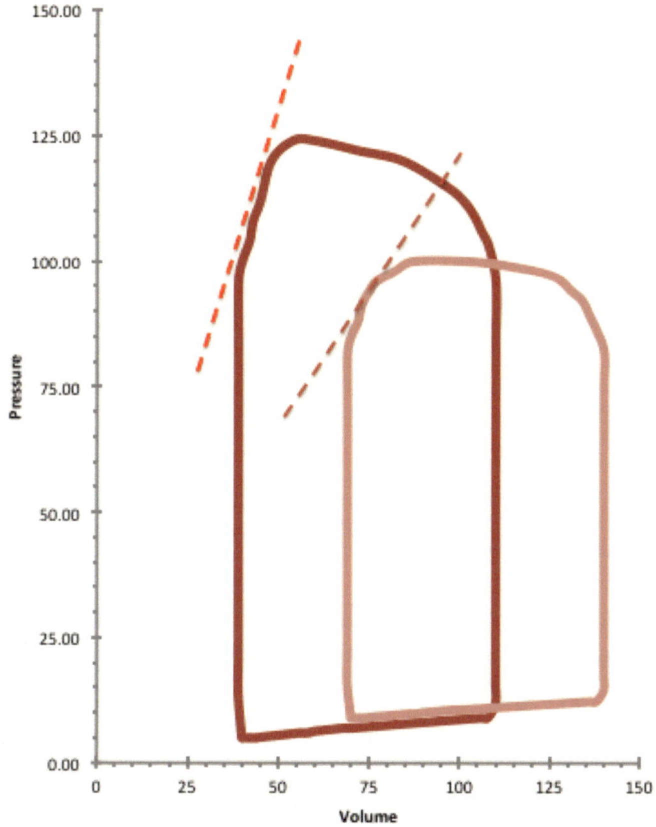

Figure 2. Pressure–volume relationship. The pressure–volume curve for the left ventricle is represented as a pressure vs. volume plot. The slope of the end-systolic pressure–volume relationship indicates the intrinsic contractile capacity of the myocardium independently of the hemodynamic load conditions. Compared to a control curve (dark lines), cardiomyopathy (light lines) is characterized by a decreased slope among other hallmarks. Gene therapy would aim at preserving or restoring normal contractility.

gene therapy, but nucleic acids can interfere in a very selective way with proteins. Targeting proteins of the intrinsic pathway of the coagulation might achieve safe and efficient thrombus control without the usual risk of bleeding that conventional anticoagulants share. Furthermore, one should keep in mind that initiation of the intrinsic pathway is intimately linked to inflammation via kinins and complement. Nucleic acid might represent a new class of drugs in this context.

Surgery represents an important therapeutic option in the arsenal for managing CM and CHF patients. The surgical approach can consist of either specific procedures such as septal myomectomy in hypertrophic CM (HCM), coronary artery bypass graft surgery, or more generally left ventricular assist devices as a "bridge to transplant" or destination therapy [24]. Transplantation remains the reference treatment for end-stage CHF and for people who have failed other treatment options. It might be surprising to refer to surgery in the context of gene therapy, but one should not forget that most initial clinical trials have included terminally ill patients. Thereby, in terms of therapeutic efficiency and risk/benefit ratio, initial evaluations will refer to outcomes of surgical procedures. The gene therapist should be aware of the competing therapeutic strategies.

So far, none of the existing treatments have definitively changed the fate of CM and CHF. There is thus space for new drug developments and gene therapy might help to solve some of the intrinsic hurdles of CM and CHF. For instance, none of the existing treatments really change myocardial contractility without excessively increasing oxygen consumption.

Advances in gene transfer vectors, development of new vector delivery methods, and discovery of new gene targets continue to fuel our motivation to use this approach in routine bedside care [25,26].

3. Gene therapy

When developing a gene therapy-based medicinal product, one should keep in mind that no active substance will become a drug product unless it can be properly formulated and administered. Compared to more conventional small molecules, gene therapy strategies based on nucleic acids are faced with new constraints linked to their chemical nature, the size of the molecule, and the coding sequence composition.

Different pharmaceutical designs for gene therapy could be considered. In the context of CM and CHF, we will focus more precisely on how to restore the functional allele in the context of inherited CM and more broadly how to restore or improve myocardial contractility.

3.1. Inherited CM

In the context of inherited CM, most frequently a monogenic transmission profile has been identified, expression profiles being either dominant or more frequently recessive. Sometimes CMs are part of a larger clinical context of a systemic myopathy, but usually cardiac and neuromuscular disorders are not proportional and thus would need separate and specific treatment, even if the genetic origin can be unique.

Considering the situation of the single causative gene acting in a recessive mode, it might be tempting to restore a normal phenotype through addition of a functional allele. So conceptually at this level, gene therapy is mainly derived from gene transfer techniques largely used in cell biology by introducing an exogenous sequence of nucleic acids into a eukaryotic cell to express new information on these cells. Over time, several independent laboratories have demonstrated that the concept of transferring an exogenous gene into the myocardium of mammals was possible, leading to the expression of a new protein not coded by the intrinsic genes. However, to transform a laboratory technique of gene transfer into a therapeutic option, additional steps had to be considered. To assess the therapeutic capabilities of gene transfer, protein expression cannot be the primary outcome measure. More subtle integration of the pathophysiology of each CM is mandatory. Considering inherited diseases where a certain phenotypic latency exists, it was possible to demonstrate that gene transfer of a functional allele was able to delay the onset of an overt CM. More generally, when designing a gene therapy strategy, one should consider whether the defective gene should be rescued or whether other genes involved in heart failure development and progression should be targeted.

3.2. Preclinical models of CM

Delta-sarcoglycan (dSG)-deficient hamsters represent a well-characterized genetically determined model of a CM. Phenotypically these animals develop a dilated cardiomyopathy (DCM) with terminal heart failure over a rather short time span as they die as mid-aged adults [27,28]. From the perspective of gene therapy they represent a very useful model. Beyond the clear phenotype, the causal genetic mutation is known, coding sequences are readily available, and transmission is autosomal recessive. A single allele correction can correct or at least clearly improve the phenotype when administered in young animals [29]. Some authors observed even more than a simple phenotypic rescue as the lifespan of these animals seemed to increase [30,31].

However, unlike dSG, coding sequences of some normal alleles can be very extensive, the most extreme case being dystrophin with a full-length cDNA of more than 11 kb. Several strategies can be considered. Given some structural specificities, reengineering of the active pharmaceutical ingredient (API) can be performed while retaining therapeutic potential. Thus, gene therapy should not simply be considered as a substitution of defective alleles. Hence, truncated forms of dystrophin have proven to alleviate pathologic phenotypes in several experiment models [32,33].

Similarly, it was possible to show that editing the intrinsic messenger RNA can lead to coding of a functional protein. Exon skipping is used to restore the reading frame within a gene. The mechanism behind exon skipping is a mutation-specific antisense oligonucleotide. An antisense oligonucleotide is a synthesized short nucleic acid polymer that will bind to the mutation site in the pre-messenger RNA to induce exon skipping. In the context of Duchenne muscular dystrophy (DMD) the genetic mutation that leads to Becker muscular dystrophy (BMD) is an in-frame deletion. Exon skipping can induce the expression of a truncated but functional dystrophin protein and thus switch the phenotype of some DMD-type mutations to the phenotype of a BMD-type mutation [34,35].

Multiple arguments in favour of the feasibility of cardiac gene therapy have been generated over time. However, these experiments raise new questions. Most non-clinical studies were carried out on well-characterized model-rescuing defective genotypes and avoiding or delaying the development of a pathological phenotype. So referring to clinical settings, this mimics mainly presymptomatic situations.

In this setting, gene therapy would basically be a prophylactic option to avoid development of a pathological phenotype, but are we ready for a gene therapy that would be mainly preventive? What would an acceptable risk/benefit ratio be in that case? Ideally in the context of preventive medicine, gene therapy of an inherited monogenic disorder should by homologous recombination correct most if not all of the affected cells without any off-target adverse effects. Gene therapy has not yet reached this level of maturity. Nevertheless, this does not mean that such options cannot be tested in the future.

3.3. Heart failure

If gene therapy offers the possibility to interfere intimately and subtly with the molecular pathways governing the pathological processes, then introducing genetic material into cells should be able not only to compensate for abnormal genes but also to influence pathways involved in the development and progression of the disease.

In the context of inherited CMs, we postulate that several steps might occur sequentially. The causative genetic defect can be inherited or be a neo-mutation and will trigger a cascade of deleterious effects that will lead to the appearance of a patent cardiac disease. Progressively the genetic features of heart failure will dominate and one might consider that at a later stage these changes will be almost independent of the original genetic defect. Moreover, we might consider that genetic modifications at this stage are similar to those that occur in the context of acquired CM. While any disease is a potential target for gene therapy, some treatments are easier to achieve in the clinic. To test this working hypothesis experimentally, we used mainly the same dSG-deficient hamster model. However, to mimic symptomatic disease, animals were included at a later age.

Many molecular targets could be considered at this level, but several candidates might be more prominent in the present context. We have already discussed the case of gene addition of a functional allele in the context of an autosomal recessive disorder. The candidate gene will of course depend on a proper identification of the genetic disease involved in the CM. On the other side, considering the heart failure phenotype as such, multiple options appear.

Rather basically, we evaluated genes preserving myocardial structure. In the experimental setting that we considered as a model, it is known that hamsters develop a DCM. However, in some substrains carrying the very same mutation but in slightly different genetic backgrounds, animals can develop firstly a phase of HCM and have a less severe phenotype. So the question became, can we mimic this feature by introducing exogenous genetic information?

Physiologic remodelling is a compensatory change in the dimensions and function of the heart in response to physiologic stimuli such as exercise and pregnancy. The remodelling process frequently includes increases in myocardial mass. The heart can respond to environmental stimuli by growth (increased myocardial mass) or shrinkage (atrophy) with a rather large dynamic range. Remodelling is induced by changes in gene expression, which, in turn, alter the expression of key regulatory proteins, the distribution and function of subcellular organelles, the size and morphology of individual cells, the properties of the extracellular matrix, and ultimately those of the entire organ. IGF-1 is a key player in this context and prior to developing a gene therapy option we could demonstrate that administration of a recombinant IGF-1 protein can exert several beneficial effects of the cardiac phenotype of dSG-deficient hamsters [36,37]. However, a recombinant protein with pleiotropic effects will inevitably lead to extracardiac adverse effects. Therefore, a gene therapy option might offer a more targeted treatment, especially when associating local delivery with tissue-specific regulatory sequences. IGF-1 served as a role model to highlight some of the innovative differences between gene therapy and conventional treatments, but of course other APIs could be developed along a similar strategy. Various pathophysiological processes could be targeted, such as interfering with the fibrosis–cell death axis and promoting cell survival.

Besides structural changes of the myocardium, influencing cardiac function could represent further targets for gene therapy strategies. Taking advantage of the well-known hamster model, one can reformulate the clinical question as the progressive decline of contractility and development of patent heart failure. We considered animals at an early symptomatic stage to mimic as closely as possible a clinically relevant situation. We compared the efficiency of administering either a functional cDNA of dSG (rescuing the causal genetic defect) or a cDNA coding for a Ca^{2+}-handling protein, for instance SERCA2a. SERCA2a holds a key role in the development and progression of heart failure, so after the initial work by Schwartz and coworkers, it was rather obvious to test its therapeutic potential [38–40]. Briefly, we could demonstrate that from a therapeutic perspective at a clinical stage of patent heart failure, great benefits could be obtained by targeting cardiomyocyte Ca^{2+} homeostasis through SERCA2a gene expression than rescuing the initial causative genetic defect [41]. These findings as well as results from several other labs strongly support the strategy of cardiac gene therapy for heart failure based on restoring appropriate Ca^{2+} handling [42–44]. At this stage, one should cite the pioneering work led by Hajjar that led to a clinical trial (CUPID) using an expression cassette coding for SERCA2a [45]. This phase IIa study retained some intrinsic limitations due to the low number of patients. Therefore, a larger phase IIb study (CUPID2) with a double-blinded, placebo-controlled, and randomized event-driven schema and based on multinational, multicenter recruitment (n = 250) was needed to confirm the initial results described in the CUPID1 study. This phase IIb CUPID2 trial did not meet its primary and secondary endpoints. Nevertheless, multiple useful data were generated by this clinical trial. Gene therapy is a realistic therapeutic strategy in the field of CMs. Patient selection is always a difficult task in those very innovative steps, but the trial allowed refining the criteria. It also became apparent how important formulation of the API and administration are. Before discussing these aspects, one should acknowledge the research done by K. Hammond and coworkers that explored the therapeutic potential of adenylyl-cyclase type 6 (AC6) [46–48]. These authors showed that activation of cardiac AC6 expression improves impaired function of aged hearts through improved calcium uptake. AC6 determines cAMP formation. However, favourable effects on cardiac function through abrogation of hypertrophy, increased cell survival, and improved calcium handling appear to be cAMP independent. The main goal of the trial based on AC6 administration in CHF patients is to evaluate the safety and efficacy of human AC6 gene product as a new therapeutic option. To reach this goal, 56 patients were (or have been if the trial is still ongoing - please check) included in this study, in which gene delivery was based on a drug formulation where human AC6 was carried by an adenovirus serotype 5.

Expression of a peptide inhibitor of GRK2 (βARKct) can improve the contractility of failing myocardium and promote reverse remodelling of the left ventricle.

Inhibition with antimiR-34a/antimiR-34 has emerged as a promising therapeutic strategy, as silencing of miR-34a attenuates cardiac dysfunction in a setting of moderate HCM. However, the beneficial effect does not appear in severe HCM [49]. Thus, it appears important to make appropriate staging of the clinical symptomatology, hence the cardiac phenotype. Therapies that inhibit miR-34a alone may have limited potential in settings of established cardiac pathology [50]. For instance, miR-133, which is enriched in cardiac and skeletal muscle, is involved in cell specification, differentiation, and development. Furthermore, miR-a33 is downregulated during cardiac hypertrophy. Specific knockdown of miR-133 via antisense targeting can be sufficient for inducing cardiac hypertrophy and reinduction of the foetal gene programme [51]. In the context of DCM it might be useful to induce a compensatory mechanism by reengaging the foetal gene programme. The miR-22 should also be considered as a critical regulator of cardiomyocyte hypertrophy and cardiac remodelling [52]. Systemic inhibition of miR-21 has proven effective against myocardial fibrosis and dysfunction [53].

Substantial advances in the understanding of the cellular and molecular basis of CMs and CHF highlight the potential utility of gene therapy as a novel therapeutic approach. However, successful clinical translation is still limited by the lack of safe, efficient, and selective delivery systems.

Naked DNA has remained the preferred method of gene delivery to the myocardium and has been explored extensively in clinical trials mainly in the setting of ischemic heart disease. The results from these trials have demonstrated efficacy with regards to secondary endpoints of reduced symptomatology, but have failed to establish significant increase in angiogenesis or an improvement in myocardial function [54].

3.4. Viral vectors for cardiac gene therapy

Viruses have evolved to become highly efficient at nucleic acid delivery to specific cell types while mostly avoiding immunosurveillance by an infected host. Several types of viruses, including retrovirus, adenovirus, adeno-associated virus (AAV), and herpes simplex virus, have been modified in the laboratory for use in gene therapy applications. Adenoviruses are an efficient gene delivery system in a broad range of cell and tissue types. However, the adverse immune reactions represent an important drawback for its development. Over time, multiple viral vector systems have been tested, but more recently AAVs have become most popular. AAVs are non-enveloped parvoviruses, which can rather easily be engineered to deliver DNA cargo to target cells. AAV vectors have demonstrated good potential for in vivo delivery of genetic material into various cells, thus appearing as a vector of choice for different therapeutic applications beyond cardiac diseases. Nevertheless, and even if some promising clinical outcomes have been reported, the current potential of viral vectors for gene therapy still faces significant restrictions, largely due to manufacturing challenges, including the absence of an efficient and scalable platform purification process [25, 55–58]. At least in the setting of murine models, AAV1, AAV6, AAV8, and AAV9 have been identified as the most cardiotropic serotypes after systemic delivery.

The concept of gene therapy seems straightforward, but this is clearly an oversimplification, and numerous problems and risks exist that prevent gene therapy using viral vectors. Due to the structure of the viral particles, AAV vectors retain limited DNA cargo capacity necessitating the need to optimize the therapeutic sequence. Multiple cells can be infected by AAVs, but overall the transduction efficiency remains low leading to increased multiplicities of infection, hence putting greater pressure on large-scale vector production. Moreover, AAVs' tropism lacks cell-type selectivity resulting in off-target transduction. Regulation of the transgene expression remains difficult and frequently results in decreased expression efficiency. Hence, to achieve optimal clinical outcome, high vector doses are required, but the presence of preexisting neutralizing antibodies precludes a number of patients from participation. Furthermore, immune elimination of infected cells often limits gene expression *in vivo*. Readministration remains a major challenge, because single shot solutions are counter-intuitive in the era of precision or personalized medicine. Further work is therefore needed to improve viral vectors, more specifically, developing stealthier AAV vectors with the aim of optimizing vector–host interactions [59–61]. Low-grade immune stimulation by the vector system appears as an important point in terms of drug development to avoid severe adverse reactions.

3.5. Non-viral vectors for cardiac gene therapy

Optimal gene therapy vectors should meet the following criteria: retaining the safety profile of naked DNA while displaying increased efficiency and decreased variability. From this perspective, non-viral methods of transfection present certain advantages such as relative ease of large-scale production, low risk of an adaptive immune response, versatility, and high safety profile.

Most of the non-viral vectors currently developed are based on polycationic molecules, which form interpolyelectrolyte complexes with the polyanionic nucleic acids. The complexes obtained generally allow for (1) efficient condensation of nucleic acids into small particles, (2) protection against degradation from nucleases, and (3) promotion of cellular uptake. These non-viral vectors usually consist of cationic lipids/liposomes (lipoplexes), cationic polymers (polyplexes), or a combination of both lipids and polymers (lipopolyplexes) [62,63].

Among these, vectors based on lipids are especially attractive due to the biocompatibility and biodegradability of lipids and phospholipids [64]. However, the toxicity displayed by cationic lipids, as well as the rapid clearance of positively charged lipoplexes, hampers further use *in vivo* of first-generation lipoplexes [64]. Coating the surface of lipoplexes, with hydrophilic polymers such as polyethylene glycol (PEG) can efficiently decrease their toxicity while increasing their circulation half-life [65]. Nonetheless, PEGylated lipoplexes often display reduced transfection efficiency due to diminished cellular uptake and can trigger anti-PEG IgM production, thus leading to accelerated blood clearance after readministration [66].

The tremendous diversity of shape, composition, and charge ratio of cationic polymers is a great asset when formulating polyplexes. Cationic polymers, which have been most widely used for cardiac gene delivery, include polyethylenimine, poly-(L-lysine), and dendrimers [67]. Despite their capacity to efficiently condense nucleic acids while preventing their degradation by nucleases and improving endosomal escape, the resulting *in vivo* gene expression remains too low and, for some of them, cytotoxic effects are detected [62,67,68].

Although non-viral vectors have dramatically improved over the past decades, they remain underrepresented for cardiac gene delivery. Further improvements to increase transfection efficiency while reducing their cytotoxicity are much needed.

From this perspective, polymers displaying few or no positive charges could be the much needed formulation for cardiac gene therapy [69]. Poloxamers, which are non-ionic amphiphilic block copolymers, were first reported by Lemieux et al. [70] as efficient formulations for muscle gene delivery. Contrary to polycationic molecules, these delivery systems do not condense DNA into small particles and display no or weak interactions with nucleic acids [69,71]. Direct intramyocardial injection of poloxamer/DNA formulations showed no toxic effect towards the myocardium although gene expression remained limited and restricted to the injection site [71]. To increase the diffusion of poloxamer/DNA formulations into the myocardium, further experiments conducted *in vivo* on larger animals, through a clinically relevant administration route, were performed. As seen in **Figure 3**, this resulted in similar gene expression rate compared to that of the same transgene delivered using an AAV1 vector. To provide more insight into poloxamer-based delivery systems, further studies addressing their mechanism of action as well as experiments evaluating the possibility to readminister these formulations should be carried out.

The principal limitation of most non-clinical studies and some clinical trials was the inability to efficiently transfer genes to the cardiac ventricles. Although *in vivo* experiments using small animals may show efficient gene transfer, many fundamental differences exist between small animal and human hearts. Large animal studies are best suited for comprehensive evaluation at the preclinical stages of therapeutic development. It might seem obvious that delivery methods should meet all criteria of clinically relevant practices. Nevertheless, some preclinical methods seem to lack this realism.

3.6. Administration strategies

With regards to the first step to translate *in vivo* gene transfer into clinically relevant gene therapy and based at least partly on the use of naked DNA, physical methods like direct intra-myocardial injections have demonstrated feasibility, but also limited efficiency. Derived from these pioneering steps, several refinements have been introduced over time. In the context of rhythm control, one should look with interest to techniques like gene painting [72]. Gene painting refers basically to an innovative technique aimed at a very

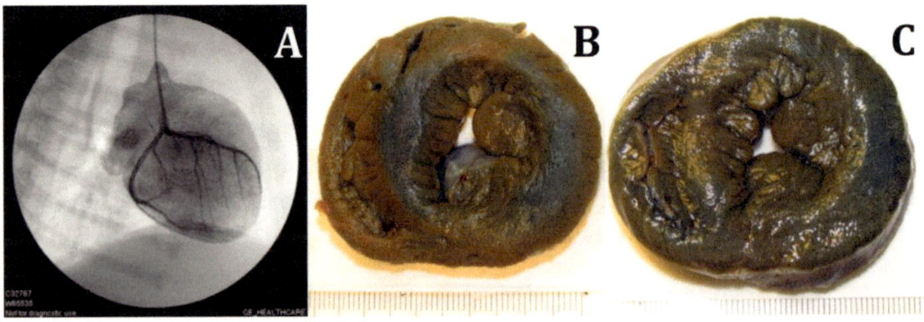

Figure 3. Preclinical evaluation of intracoronary vector administration in large animals, for instance Beagle dogs. Similar amounts of cDNA were formulated differently. (A) Sample of a coronary contrast injection of the left main coronary artery in a dog heart highlighting the route of administration. (B) Mid-ventricular cross-section after AAV1 vectorization of a lacZ coding cDNA. (C) Mid-ventricular cross-section after polymer P85 vectorization of a lacZ coding cDNA. X-gal staining reveals lacZ gene expression (unpublished results).

local gene transfer by a topical administration. Proof-of-concept studies have shown the efficiency of this approach in atrial fibrillation. Strategies based on ultrasound-targeted microbubble destruction could be a promising method for gene delivery [73]. Microbubbles are small (<5 μm) gas-filled voids that are generally stabilized by phospholipids or synthetic polymers. The use of microbubbles as gene vectors is based on the paradigm that destruction of the DNA-loaded microbubbles by ultrasounds will result in local transduction and still spare non-target areas. Percutaneous antegrade coronary injections are among the least invasive cardiac selective gene delivery methods and are rather broadly available. Intracoronary delivery allows diffuse transduction throughout the myocardium, but as such it is a highly inefficient process. However, dense regional gene transfer (>80% of myocytes in the target territory) is possible. Pharmacological manipulations to induce vasodilation and maximize vascular permeability in a specific coronary perfusion territory can greatly improve transfection efficiency [74]. Given the high perfusion velocity and the submaximal extent of the vascular bed, one has to maximize the duration of vector exposure to the local vasculature while minimizing the systemic distribution. Several options have been tested such as pharmacologically induced coronary artery dilation, blocking the venous return or developing a cardiac recirculation approach. Delivery methods based on cardiopulmonary bypass (CPB) with a closed-loop system can be used for cardiac gene therapy [75,76]. It might seem excessive to selectively prescribe CPB for gene delivery given the clearly invasive nature of such a procedure. Nevertheless, one should not forget that many of the CM/heart failure patients might need invasive procedures due to their clinical condition. Gene therapy should also be evaluated in the context of combination therapies. CM/heart failure presents as a syndrome with multiple pathophysiological facets. Early treatment of some specific aspects like atrial fibrillation by gene therapy might be as efficient as conventional cardioversion. Targeting the autonomous nervous system through gene therapy should be evaluated with reference to current beta-blockers. Inotropism might be improved by means of additive gene therapy, for example. However, beyond the diversity of gene therapy targets, combination with more conventional drugs might be improved by reinforcing the target pathways.

4. Conclusions

Gene therapy is emerging as a suitable alternative, with substantial progress in preclinical models of cardiovascular disorders. Despite the fact that none of the clinical trials, which investigated new treatments for CMs, has met their primary efficacy endpoints, subanalysis, however, has demonstrated potential efficacy. Inadequate gene delivery remains one of the underlying causes behind failures seen in clinical trials. Higher transduction efficiency is needed to achieve therapeutic effects. Use of block copolymers in gene delivery is a promising area of research, in which new and important developments are expected.

CMs can serve as a disease model for several aspects when it comes to the development of gene therapy strategies in the context of cardiac diseases, since they also engulf inherited diseases like acquired disorders.

The emphasis on gene therapies was initially focused on inherited diseases notably rescuing cardiac phenotype by introducing a functional allele in the context of recessive disorders. Even gene therapies that would only help a couple of thousand people would be a remarkable achievement.

More recently the concept of gene therapy has been extended to a larger perspective, including the reprogramming of failing myocardial cells beyond inherited diseases. Several non-clinical studies have supported the concept, but the true challenge of gene therapy for CM remains translation into the clinic. Sticking to the old paradigm that a drug substance can only become a medicinal drug product, if one is able to formulate and administer it, it seems more obvious that gene therapy has to be clinically oriented. Treating the failing heart implies several strong constraints linked to the anatomy and physiology of the heart. Successful gene therapy approaches in other diseases support the notion, but cannot fully address the underlying specific challenges facing cardiac gene delivery.

The development of robust administration techniques and improved formulations are therefore needed before cardiac gene therapy can be integrated into the therapeutic armamentarium.

Acknowledgments

The authors are grateful to the late Ketty Schwartz and Marc Fiszman for their great mentorship and for developing a cardiac gene therapy programme at the very early stage of the field.

Conflict of interest

The authors declare no conflict of interest.

Author details

Yves Fromes[1*] and Caroline Roques[2,3,4,5]

*Address all correspondence to: yves.fromes@gmail.com

1 UPMC, Sorbonne Universities, Institute of Myology, Paris, France

2 Université Paris Descartes, Sorbonne-Paris-Cité, UTCBS, Paris, France

3 CNRS, UTCBS UMR 8258, Paris, France

4 Chimie ParisTech, PSL Research University, Unité de Technologies Chimiques et Biologiques pour la Santé (UTCBS), Paris, France

5 INSERM, UTCBS U 1022, Paris, France

References

[1] Sen-Chowdhry S, McKenna WJ. Sudden death from genetic and acquired cardiomyopathies. Circulation. 2012;**125**:1563-1576

[2] Nakamura A. X-linked dilated cardiomyopathy: A cardiospecific phenotype of dystrophinopathy. Pharmaceuticals. 2015;**8**(2):303-320

[3] Kamdar F, Garry DJ. Dystrophin-deficient cardiomyopathy. Journal of the American College of Cardiology. 2016;**67**:2533-2546

[4] Niimura H, Patton KK, McKenna WJ, Soults J, Maron BJ, Seidman JG, et al. Sarcomere protein gene mutations in hypertrophic cardiomyopathy of the elderly. Circulation. 2002;**105**:446-451

[5] Finsterer J, Stöllberger C. Unclassified cardiomyopathies in neuromuscular disorders. Wiener Medizinische Wochenschrift. 2013;**163**:505-513

[6] Finsterer J, Stöllberger C, Wahbi K. Cardiomyopathy in neurological disorders. Cardiovascular Pathology. 2013;**22**:389-400

[7] Yoshikawa T. Contribution of acquired factors to the pathogenesis of dilated cardiomyopathy. The cause of dilated cardiomyopathy: Genetic or acquired? (acquired-side). Circulation Journal. 2011;**75**:1766-1773; discussion 1773

[8] O'Hanlon R, Mohiaddin RH. Inherited cardiomyopathies. In: Magnetic Resonance Imaging of Congenital Heart Disease. Springer-Verlag London Ltd; 2012. pp. 211-229

[9] O'Hanlon R, Assomull RG, Prasad SK. Use of cardiovascular magnetic resonance for diagnosis and management in hypertrophic cardiomyopathy. Current Cardiology Reports. 2007;**9**:51-56

[10] Saito S, Tanoue M, Masuda K, Mori Y, Nakatani S, Yoshioka Y, et al. Longitudinal observations of progressive cardiac dysfunction in a cardiomyopathic animal model by self-gated cine imaging based on 11.7-T magnetic resonance imaging. Scientific Reports. 2017;**7**(1):1-10

[11] Shehata ML, Turkbey EB, Vogel-Claussen J, Bluemke DA. Role of cardiac magnetic resonance imaging in assessment of nonischemic cardiomyopathies. Topics in Magnetic Resonance Imaging. 2008;**19**(1):43-57

[12] Haaf P, Garg P, Messroghli DR, Broadbent DA, Greenwood JP, Plein S. Cardiac T1 mapping and extracellular volume (ECV) in clinical practice: A comprehensive review. Journal of Cardiovascular Magnetic Resonance. 2016;**18**:1-12

[13] Fraysse B, Nagi SM, Boher B, Ragot H, Lainé J, Salmon A, et al. Ca^{2+} overload and mitochondrial permeability transition pore activation in living-sarcoglycan-deficient cardiomyocytes. American Journal of Physiology. Cell Physiology. 2010;**299**:C706-C713

[14] Ghonim S, Voges I, Gatehouse PD, Keegan J, Gatzoulis MA, Kilner PJ, et al. Myocardial architecture, mechanics, and fibrosis in congenital heart disease. Frontiers in Cardiovascular Medicine. 2017;**4**:303389-303330

[15] Schirone L, Forte M, Palmerio S, Yee D, Nocella C, Angelini F, et al. A review of the molecular mechanisms underlying the development and progression of cardiac remodeling. Oxidative Medicine and Cellular Longevity. 2017;**2017**:1-16

[16] Karamitsos T, Neubauer S. Cardiovascular magnetic resonance imaging. Medicine (Baltimore). 2014;**42**:461-467

[17] Ridker PM. Targeting inflammatory pathways for the treatment of cardiovascular disease. European Heart Journal. 2014;**35**:540-543

[18] Ridker PM, Everett BM, Thuren T, MacFadyen JG, Chang WH, Ballantyne C, et al. Antiinflammatory therapy with canakinumab for atherosclerotic disease. The New England Journal of Medicine. 2017;**377**(12):1191-1131

[19] Van Tassell BW, Canada J, Carbone S, Trankle C, Buckley L, Oddi Erdle C, et al. Interleukin-1 blockade in recently decompensated systolic heart failure. Circulation: Heart Failure. 2017;**10**:e004373

[20] Heinrich PC, Behrmann I, Müller-Newen G, Schaper F, Graeve L. Interleukin-6-type cytokine signalling through the gp130/Jak/STAT pathway. The Biochemical Journal. 1998;**334**:297-314

[21] Fischer P, Hilfiker-Kleiner D. Role of gp130-mediated signalling pathways in the heart and its impact on potential therapeutic aspects. British Journal of Pharmacology. 2008;**153**:S414-S427

[22] Ritschel VN, Seljeflot I, Arnesen H, Halvorsen S, Eritsland J, Fagerland MW, et al. Circulating levels of IL-6 receptor and gp130 and long-term clinical outcomes in ST-elevation myocardial infarction. Journal of the American Heart Association. 2016;**5**(6):1-8

[23] Hilfiker-Kleiner D, Shukla P, Klein G, Schaefer A, Stapel B, Hoch M, et al. Continuous glycoprotein-130-mediated signal transducer and activator of transcription-3 activation promotes inflammation, left ventricular rupture, and adverse outcome in subacute myocardial infarction. Circulation. 2010;**122**:145-155

[24] Schmidt M, Burrell A, Roberts L, Bailey M, Sheldrake J, Rycus PT, et al. Predicting survival after ECMO for refractory cardiogenic shock: The survival after veno-arterial-ECMO (SAVE)-score. European Heart Journal. 2015;**36**:2246-2256

[25] Hammoudi N, Ishikawa K, Hajjar RJ. Adeno-associated virus-mediated gene therapy in cardiovascular disease. Current Opinion in Cardiology. 2015;**30**:228-234

[26] Rincon MY, VandenDriessche T, Chuah MK. Gene therapy for cardiovascular disease: Advances in vector development, targeting, and delivery for clinical translation. Cardiovascular Research. 2015;**108**:4-20

[27] Fromes Y, Parzy E, Carlier P, Fiszman MY. In vivo evaluation of the cardiac disease in myopathic hamster strain CHF147. Journal of Molecular and Cellular Cardiology. 2002;**34**:A23

[28] Parzy E, Fromes Y, Thiaudiere E, Carlier PG. Refinement of cardiac NMR imaging in awake hamsters: Proof of feasibility and characterization of cardiomyopathy. NMR in Biomedicine. 2007;**20**:615-623

[29] Holt KH, Lim LE, Straub V, Venzke DP, Duclos F, Anderson RD, et al. Functional rescue of the sarcoglycan complex in the BIO 14.6 hamster using delta-sarcoglycan gene transfer. Molecular Cell. 1998;**1**:841-848

[30] Li J, Wang D, Qian S, Chen Z, Zhu T, Xiao X. Efficient and long-term intracardiac gene transfer in delta-sarcoglycan-deficiency hamster by adeno-associated virus-2 vectors. Gene Therapy. 2003;**10**:1807-1813

[31] Hoshijima M. Delta-sarcoglycan gene therapy halts progression of cardiac dysfunction, improves respiratory failure and prolongs life in myopathic hamsters. Circulation. 2011;**4**:89-97

[32] Shin J-H, Pan X, Hakim CH, Yang HT, Yue Y, Zhang K, et al. Microdystrophin ameliorates muscular dystrophy in the canine model of Duchenne muscular dystrophy. Molecular Therapy. 2013;**21**:750-757

[33] Le Guiner C, Servais L, Montus M, Larcher T, Fraysse B, Moullec S, et al. Long-term microdystrophin gene therapy is effective in a canine model of Duchenne muscular dystrophy. Nature Communications. 2017;**8**:16105

[34] Vulin A, Barthélémy I, Goyenvalle A, Thibaud J-L, Beley C, Griffith G, et al. Muscle function recovery in golden retriever muscular dystrophy after AAV1-U7 exon skipping. Molecular Therapy. 2012;**20**:2120-2133

[35] Goyenvalle A, Griffith G, Babbs A, Andaloussi SE, Ezzat K, Avril A, et al. Functional correction in mouse models of muscular dystrophy using exon-skipping tricyclo-DNA oligomers. Nature Medicine. 2015;**21**(3):270-275

[36] Serose A, Prudhon B, Salmon AA, Doyennette MAA, Fiszman MY, Fromes Y. Administration of insulin-like growth factor-1 (IGF-1) improves both structure and function of delta-sarcoglycan deficient cardiac muscle in the hamster. Basic Research in Cardiology. 2005;**100**:161-170

[37] Serose A, Salmon AA, Fiszman MY, Fromes Y. Short-term treatment using insulin-like growth factor-1 (IGF-1) improves life expectancy of the delta-sarcoglycan deficient hamster. Journal Genetics in Medicine. 2006;**8**:1048-1055

[38] Ribadeau Dumas A, Wisnewsky C, Boheler KR, Ter Keurs H, Fiszman MY, Schwartz K. The sarco(endo)plasmic reticulum Ca(2+)-ATPase gene is regulated at the transcriptional level during compensated left ventricular hypertrophy in the rat. Comptes Rendus de l'Académie des Sciences. Série III. 1997;**320**:963-969

[39] Ribadeau-Dumas A, Brady M, Boateng SY, Schwartz K, Boheler KR. Sarco(endo)plasmic reticulum Ca(2+)-ATPase (SERCA2) gene products are regulated post-transcriptionally during rat cardiac development. Cardiovascular Research. 1999;**43**:426-436

[40] Arai M. SERCA2 as a cause and therapeutic target of heart failure. Folia Pharmacologica Japonica. 2012;**140**:259-264

[41] Bouyon S, Roussel V, Fromes Y. SERCA2a gene therapy can improve symptomatic heart failure in δ-sarcoglycan-deficient animals. Human Gene Therapy. 2014;**25**:694-704

[42] Gwathmey JK, Yerevanian AI, Hajjar RJ. Cardiac gene therapy with SERCA2a: From bench to bedside. Journal of Molecular and Cellular Cardiology. 2011;**50**:803-812

[43] Hajjar RJ. Potential of gene therapy as a treatment for heart failure. The Journal of Clinical Investigation. 2013;**123**:53-61

[44] Fish KM, Ishikawa K. Advances in gene therapy for heart failure. Discovery Medicine. 2015;**19**:285-291

[45] Kratlian RG, Hajjar RJ. Cardiac gene therapy: From concept to reality. Current Heart Failure Reports. 2012;**9**:33-39

[46] Tang T, Hammond HK, Firth A, Yang Y, Gao MH, Yuan JX-J, et al. Adenylyl cyclase 6 improves calcium uptake and left ventricular function in aged hearts. Journal of the American College of Cardiology. 2011;**57**:1846-1855

[47] Gao MH, Tang T, Lai NC, Miyanohara A, Guo T, Tang R, et al. Beneficial effects of adenylyl cyclase type 6 (AC6) expression persist using a catalytically inactive AC6 mutant. Molecular Pharmacology. 2011;**79**:381-388

[48] Gao MH, Hammond HK. Unanticipated signaling events associated with cardiac adenylyl cyclase gene transfer. Journal of Molecular and Cellular Cardiology. 2011;**50**:751-758

[49] Bernardo BC, Gao X-M, Winbanks CE, Boey EJH, Tham YK, Kiriazis H, et al. Therapeutic inhibition of the miR-34 family attenuates pathological cardiac remodeling and improves heart function. Proceedings of the National Academy of Sciences. 2012;**109**:17615-17620

[50] Bernardo BC, Gao XM, Tham YK, Kiriazis H, Winbanks CE, Ooi JYY, et al. Silencing of miR-34a attenuates cardiac dysfunction in a setting of moderate, but not severe, hypertrophic cardiomyopathy. PLoS One. 2014;**9**(2):e90337

[51] Abdellatif M. The role of miR-133 in cardiac hypertrophy uncovered. Cardiovascular Research. 2011;**106**:16-18

[52] Huang ZP, Chen J, Seok HY, Zhang Z, Kataoka M, Hu X, et al. MicroRNA-22 regulates cardiac hypertrophy and remodeling in response to stress. Circulation Research. 2013;**112**:1234-1243

[53] Duygu B, Da Costa Martins PA. MiR-21: A star player in cardiac hypertrophy. Cardiovascular Research. 2015;**105**:235-237

[54] Shah PB, Losordo DW. Non-viral vectors for gene therapy: Clinical trials in cardiovascular disease. Advances in Genetics. 2005;**54**:339-361

[55] Berns KI, Muzyczka N. AAV: An overview of unanswered questions. Human Gene Therapy. 2017;**28**:308-313

[56] Servais L, Le Guiner C, Montus M, Cherel Y, Francois CJ, Thibaud JL, et al. Persistence and stability at 6 months of AAV genome and dystrophin expression in GRMD dogs after forelimb delivery of a recombinant AAV carrying an exon skipping sequence. Neuromuscular Disorders. 2014;**24**:822

[57] Naso MF, Tomkowicz B, Perry WL, Strohl WR. Adeno-associated virus (AAV) as a vector for gene therapy. BioDrugs. 2017;**31**:317-334

[58] Grieger JC, Samulski RJ. Adeno-associated virus as a gene therapy vector: Vector development, production and clinical applications. Advances in Biochemical Engineering/Biotechnology. 2005;**99**:119-145

[59] Buning H, Huber A, Zhang L, Meumann N, Hacker U. Engineering the AAV capsid to optimize vector-host-interactions. Current Opinion in Pharmacology. 2015;**24**:94-104

[60] Selot RS, Hareendran S, Jayandharan GR. Developing immunologically inert adeno-associated virus (AAV) vectors for gene therapy: Possibilities and limitations. Current Pharmaceutical Biotechnology. 2014;**14**:1072-1082

[61] Ertl HC, High KA. The impact of AAV capsid-specific T cell responses on design and outcome of clinical gene transfer trials with recombinant AAV vectors—An evolving controversy. Human Gene Therapy. 2017;**28**(4):328-337

[62] Goodwin T, Huang L. Nonviral vectors: We have come a long way. Advances in Genetics. 2014;**88**:1-12

[63] Guan S, Rosenecker J. Nanotechnologies in delivery of mRNA therapeutics using nonviral vector-based delivery systems. Gene Therapy. 2017;**24**:133-143

[64] Xue HY, Guo P, Wen W-C, Wong HL. Lipid-based nanocarriers for RNA delivery. Current Pharmaceutical Design. 2015;**21**:3140-3147

[65] Harvie P, Wong FMP, Bally MB. Use of poly (ethylene glycol)–lipid conjugates to regulate the surface attributes and transfection activity of lipid–DNA particles. Journal of Pharmaceutical Sciences. 2000;**89**:652-663

[66] Tagami T, Uehara Y, Moriyoshi N, Ishida T, Kiwada H. Anti-PEG IgM production by siRNA encapsulated in a PEGylated lipid nanocarrier is dependent on the sequence of the siRNA. Journal of Controlled Release. 2011;**151**:149-154

[67] Su C-H, Wu Y-J, Wang H-H, Yeh H-I. Nonviral gene therapy targeting cardiovascular system. American Journal of Physiology: Heart and Circulatory Physiology. 2012;**303**:H629-H638

[68] Roques C, Salmon A, Fiszman MY, Fattal E, Fromes Y. Intrapericardial administration of novel DNA formulations based on thermosensitive Poloxamer 407 gel. International Journal of Pharmaceutics. 2007;**331**:220-223

[69] Roques C, Fromes Y, Fattal E. Hydrosoluble polymers for muscular gene delivery. European Journal of Pharmaceutics and Biopharmaceutics. 2009;**72**:378-390

[70] Lemieux P, Guérin N, Paradis G, Proulx R, Chistyakova L, Kabanov A, et al. A combination of poloxamers increases gene expression of plasmid DNA in skeletal muscle. Gene Therapy. 2000;**7**:986-991

[71] Roques C, Fattal E, Fromes Y. Comparison of toxicity and transfection efficiency of amphiphilic block copolymers and polycationic polymers in striated muscles. Journal of Genetics in Medicine. 2009;**11**:240-249

[72] Liu Z, Donahue JK. The use of gene therapy for ablation of atrial fibrillation. Arrhythmia & Electrophysiology Review. 2014;**3**:139-144

[73] Liu Y, Li L, Su Q, Liu T, Ma Z, Yang H. Ultrasound-targeted microbubble destruction enhances gene expression of microRNA-21 in swine heart via intracoronary delivery. Echocardiography. 2015;**32**:1407-1416

[74] Sasano T, Kikuchi K, McDonald AD, Lai S, Donahue JK. Targeted high-efficiency, homogeneous myocardial gene transfer. Journal of Molecular and Cellular Cardiology. 2007;**42**:954-961

[75] Swain JD, Katz MG, White JD, Thesier DM, Henderson A, Stedman HH, et al. A translatable, closed recirculation system for AAV6 vector-mediated myocardial gene delivery in the large animal. Methods in Molecular Biology. 2011;**709**:331-354

[76] Katz MG, Fargnoli AS, Weber T, Hajjar R, Bridges C. Use of Adeno-associated virus vector for cardiac gene delivery in large animal surgical models of heart failure. Human Gene Therapy. Clinical Development. 2017;**28**(3):157-164